AF412797

Advances in Oto-Rhino-Laryngology

Vol. 76

Series Editor

G. Randolph Boston, Mass.

Surgery for Pediatric Velopharyngeal Insufficiency

Volume Editors

Nikhila Raol Boston, Mass.

Christopher J. Hartnick Boston, Mass.

34 figures, 25 in color, 1 table, 2015

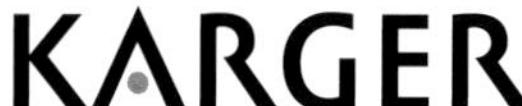

KARGER

Basel · Freiburg · Paris · London · New York · Chennai · New Delhi ·
Bangkok · Beijing · Shanghai · Tokyo · Kuala Lumpur · Singapore · Sydney

Nikhila Raol
Fellow, Pediatric Otolaryngology
Massachusetts Eye and Ear Infirmary
243 Charles St.
Boston, MA 02114 (USA)

Christopher J. Hartnick
Chief, Pediatric Otolaryngology
Massachusetts Eye and Ear Infirmary
243 Charles St.
Boston, MA 02114 (USA)

Library of Congress Cataloging-in-Publication Data

Surgery for pediatric velopharyngeal insufficiency / volume editors, Nikhila
Raol, Christopher J. Hartnick.
    p. ; cm. -- (Advances in oto-rhino-laryngology, ISSN 0065-3071 ;
vol. 76)
  Includes bibliographical references and indexes.
  ISBN 978-3-318-02786-0 (hard cover : alk. paper) -- ISBN 978-3-318-02787-7
(electronic version)
  I. Raol, Nikhila, editor. II. Hartnick, Christopher J., editor. III.
Series: Advances in oto-rhino-laryngology ; v. 76. 0065-3071
  [DNLM: 1. Velopharyngeal Insufficiency--surgery. 2. Child. W1 AD701
v.76 2015 / WV 410]
  RF497.V84
  617.5'32--dc23

                      2014044357

Bibliographic Indices. This publication is listed in bibliographic services, including Current Contents®.

Disclaimer. The statements, opinions and data contained in this publication are solely those of the individual authors and contributors and not of the publisher and the editor(s). The appearance of advertisements in the book is not a warranty, endorsement, or approval of the products or services advertised or of their effectiveness, quality or safety. The publisher and the editor(s) disclaim responsibility for any injury to persons or property resulting from any ideas, methods, instructions or products referred to in the content or advertisements.

Drug Dosage. The authors and the publisher have exerted every effort to ensure that drug selection and dosage set forth in this text are in accord with current recommendations and practice at the time of publication. However, in view of ongoing research, changes in government regulations, and the constant flow of information relating to drug therapy and drug reactions, the reader is urged to check the package insert for each drug for any change in indications and dosage and for added warnings and precautions. This is particularly important when the recommended agent is a new and/or infrequently employed drug.

All rights reserved. No part of this publication may be translated into other languages, reproduced or utilized in any form or by any means electronic or mechanical, including photocopying, recording, microcopying, or by any information storage and retrieval system, without permission in writing from the publisher.

© Copyright 2015 by S. Karger AG, P.O. Box, CH-4009 Basel (Switzerland)
www.karger.com
Printed in Germany on acid-free and non-aging paper (ISO 9706) by Kraft Druck GmbH, Ettlingen
ISSN 0065–3071
e-ISSN 1662–2847
ISBN 978–3–318–02786–0
e-ISBN 978–3–318–02787–7

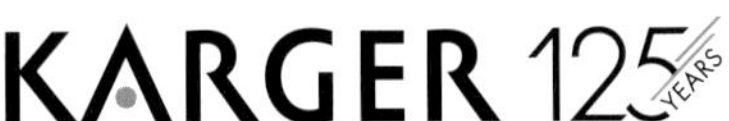

Contents

Online supplementary material: www.karger.com/adorl076_suppl

Preface

Our book, '*Surgery for Pediatric Velopharyngeal Insufficiency*,' was a concept that was born out of a simple search for instructional videos for velopharyngeal insufficiency (VPI) surgery for new trainees. Realizing how helpful it is to see the operation in addition to reading the steps, we came up with a textbook that is truly designed for surgeons who treat VPI or who are interested in learning how to treat VPI.

The textbook describes the multidisciplinary approach to pediatric VPI, describing the roles of the speech pathologist, radiologist, and prosthodontist. However, our main goal was to create a book for the surgeon, highlighting important surgical concepts, both through text and audiovisual media, that are essential for the successful treatment of VPI.

We hope that you find this book both enjoyable to read and helpful in your practice. We would like to thank our families for their support and patience, our colleagues for their input and always-pleasant nature, and our patients for allowing us to play a small role in their lives.

Nikhila Raol, MD, Boston, Mass., USA
Christopher J. Hartnick, MD, MS Epi., Boston, Mass., USA

Raol N, Hartnick CJ (eds): Surgery for Pediatric Velopharyngeal Insufficiency.
Adv Otorhinolaryngol. Basel, Karger, 2015, vol 76, pp 1–6 (DOI: 10.1159/000368003)

Anatomy and Physiology of Velopharyngeal Closure and Insufficiency

Nikhila Raol · Christopher J. Hartnick

Fellow, Pediatric Otolaryngology, Massachusetts Eye and Ear Infirmary, Boston, Mass., USA

Abstract

The velopharynx is a complex structure that is responsible for separation of the oral and nasal cavities during speech production and swallowing. Incompetence of this mechanism can lead to hypernasality, with nasal air emission and incomprehensible speech, as well as nasopharyngeal regurgitation. There can be a significant social stigma associated with velopharyngeal dysfunction, and surgical treatment can be curative in many cases. Knowledge of the normal anatomy and physiology of the velopharyngeal complex is essential when planning for surgical repair.

© 2015 S. Karger AG, Basel

Anatomy

The velopharyngeal sphincter is bounded anteriorly by the soft palate, or velum; laterally by the lateral pharyngeal walls; and posteriorly by the posterior pharyngeal wall. It is composed of six muscle types: the levator veli palatini, tensor veli palatini, musculus uvulae, palatoglossus, palatopharyngeus, and superior pharyngeal constrictor (fig. 1). The levator veli palatini originates from the inferior surface of the petrous portion of the temporal bone and the medial rim of the Eustachian tube. The muscles take an anterior, inferior, and medial course to then decussate with the fibers of the contralateral levator muscle at the palatine aponeurosis in the midline. The levator sling makes up the majority of the muscle mass in the palate, and its orientation and function are essential for proper velopharyngeal function.

The tensor veli palatini originates from the medial pterygoid plate and from the lateral rim of the Eustachian tube. It runs anterior and lateral to the levator and ends

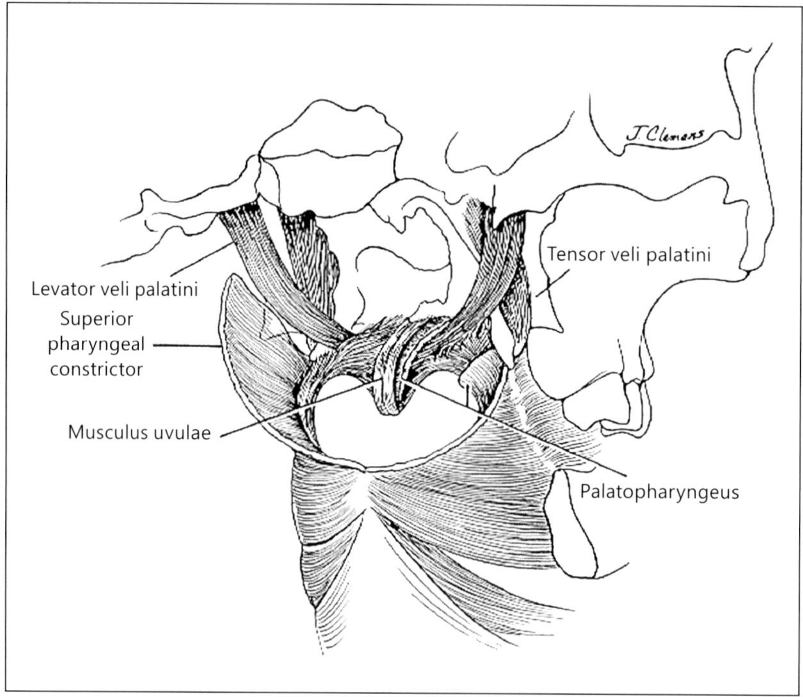

Fig. 1. Velopharyngeal muscular anatomy. Reprinted with permission from Bluestone's Pediatric Otolaryngology, 4th edition.

in a tendon that wraps around the pterygoid hamulus of the sphenoid bone and inserts into the palatine aponeurosis. Its primary function is to tense the soft palate and thereby assist the levator veli palatini in uncoupling the oral and nasal cavities. The tensor veli palatini is innervated by the medial pterygoid nerve, a branch of the mandibular nerve, which is itself the third division of the trigeminal nerve. This makes it the only muscle involved in the velopharyngeal mechanism that is not innervated by the vagus nerve. Surgically, the tensor veli palatini can be important in helping with tension-free closure in palatoplasty. In cases of Furlow palatoplasty, increased laxity can be obtained for closure by infracturing the hamulus around which the tensor tendon passes. The hamulus can be palpated as a bilateral symmetric bony bump that is slightly medial to the maxillary tuberosity at the junction of the hard and soft palates. Although hamulus fracture is not frequently performed, it is a good adjunct technique to be aware of in cases of difficult palate closure.

The musculus uvulae are paired intrinsic muscles that arise from the posterior nasal spine of the palatine bones and from the palatine aponeurosis and insert into the uvula. They are thought to aid in velopharyngeal closure by increasing the midline bulk and by extending the length of the nasal aspect of the velum, thus maximizing apposition of the soft palate to the posterior pharyngeal wall [1]. In patients with a cleft palate or a submucosal cleft, these muscles are typically deficient [2]. The triad of a bifid uvula, palatal notching, and soft palate diastasis should alert the surgeon to a high likelihood of a submucosal cleft, and in these cases, only superior adenoidectomy should be performed. The risk of velopharyngeal insufficiency (VPI) following adenoidectomy is approximately 1:1,500, and the risk is higher in patients with a submucosal cleft palate.

The palatoglossus, also known as the anterior tonsillar pillar, originates in the anterior soft palate, where it is continuous with the contralateral muscle and courses laterally, inferiorly, and anteriorly to insert into the tongue. The palatopharyngeus, or the posterior tonsillar pillar, originates in the soft palate as well and passes laterally, inferiorly, and posteriorly to join the stylopharyngeus and insert into the posterior border of the thyroid cartilage. Both of these muscles depress the palate, hence creating an opposing force to the action of the levator veli palatini. They are thought to provide fine motor control of the soft palate position while speaking [3]. It is important to note the impact of aggressive resection of the palatopharyngeus during a tonsillectomy, as scarring in this area can lead to tethering of the soft palate and subsequent VPI.

The superior pharyngeal constrictor is made up of four parts: pterygopharyngeal (origin: medial pterygoid), buccopharyngeal (origin: pterygomandibular raphe), mylopharyngeal (origin: mandible above mylohyoid line), and glossopharyngeal (origin: tongue) parts. Despite different origins, all of these parts join and decussate with contralateral fibers to insert into the median pharyngeal raphe. The primary function of the constrictor muscle is medial displacement of the lateral pharyngeal walls and some anterior displacement of the posterior pharyngeal wall, thereby narrowing the velopharyngeal port and allowing for improved contact between the soft palate and the posterior pharyngeal wall [4]. From a surgical standpoint, it is important to note that due to the significant redundancy of this muscle, the posterior pharyngeal wall can be easily closed primarily when tissue is borrowed for a pharyngeal flap or for a sphincter pharyngoplasty.

In approximately 20% of the population, a bulge along the posterior pharyngeal wall due to contraction of the superior pharyngeal constrictor may be seen. First described in 1863 by Passavant and therefore termed Passavant's ridge, it is believed by some to aid in velopharyngeal closure, although this is controversial [5].

Normal Physiology

In individuals with a normal velopharyngeal mechanism, contraction primarily of the levator veli palatini causes the velum to move superiorly and posteriorly, contacting the posterior pharyngeal wall and closing the velopharyngeal port. The site and extent of contact depend on the sound that is being produced [6, 7]. This description is rather simplistic, however; the actual closure pattern is based on the variable participation of the muscles described above.

Pearls and Pitfalls

Knowledge of normal velopharyngeal anatomy and closure patterns is imperative for accurate surgical decision-making.

Velopharyngeal mislearning should be recognized early so as to prevent unnecessary surgery or to convey realistic expectations for surgery when multiple types of velopharyngeal dysfunction are present.

References

1 Huang MH, Lee ST, Rajendran K: Structure of the musculus uvulae: functional and surgical implications of an anatomic study. Cleft Palate Craniofac J 1997;34:466–474.

2 Lewin ML, Croft CB, Shprintzen RJ: Velopharyngeal insufficiency due to hypoplasia of the musculus uvulae and occult submucous cleft palate. Plast Reconstr Surg 1980;65:585–591.

3 Moon JB, Smith AE, Folkins JW, Lemke JH, Gartlan M: Coordination of velopharyngeal muscle activity during positioning of the soft palate. Cleft Palate Craniofac J 1994;31:45–55.

4 Shprintzen RJ, McCall GN, Skolnick ML, Lencione RM: Selective movement of the lateral aspects of the pharyngeal walls during velopharyngeal closure for speech, blowing, and whistling in normals. Cleft Palate J 1975;12:51–58.

5 Ruda JM, Krakovitz P, Rose AS: A review of the evaluation and management of velopharyngeal insufficiency in children. Otolaryngol Clin North Am 2012;45:653–669, viii.

6 Moll KL: Velopharyngeal closure on vowels. J Speech Hear Res 1962;5:30–37.

7 Karnell MP, Linville RN, Edwards BA: Variations in velar position over time: a nasal videoendoscopic study. J Speech Hear Res 1988;31:417–424.

8 Skolnick ML, McCall GN, Barnes M: The sphincteric mechanism of velopharyngeal closure. Cleft Palate J 1973;10:286–305.

9 Ruotolo RA, Veitia NA, Corbin A, et al: Velopharyngeal anatomy in 22q11.2 deletion syndrome: a three-dimensional cephalometric analysis. Cleft Palate Craniofac J 2006;43:446–456.

10 Shprintzen RJ, Sher AE, Croft CB: Hypernasal speech caused by tonsillar hypertrophy. Int J Pediatr Otorhinolaryngol 1987;14:45–56.

11 Johns DF, Rohrich RJ, Awada M: Velopharyngeal incompetence: a guide for clinical evaluation. Plast Reconstr Surg 2003;112:1890–1897; quiz 1898, 1982.

12 McHenry MA: Aerodynamic, acoustic, and perceptual measures of nasality following traumatic brain injury. Brain Inj 1999;13:281–290.

13 Duffy JR: Stroke with dysarthria: evaluate and treat; garden variety or down the garden path? Semin Speech Lang 1998;19:93–98; quiz 99.

14 Peterson-Falzone SJ, Graham MS: Phoneme-specific nasal emission in children with and without physical anomalies of the velopharyngeal mechanism. J Speech Hear Disord 1990;55:132–139.

15 Shriberg LD, Aram DM, Kwiatkowski J: Developmental apraxia of speech: I. Descriptive and theoretical perspectives. J Speech Lang Hear Res 1997;40:273–285.

16 Trost JE: Articulatory additions to the classical description of the speech of persons with cleft palate. Cleft Palate J 1981;18:193–203.

17 Dworkin JP, Marunick MT, Krouse JH: Velopharyngeal dysfunction: speech characteristics, variable etiologies, evaluation techniques, and differential treatments. Lang Speech Hear Serv Sch 2004;35:333–352.

Christopher J. Hartnick, MD
Chief, Pediatric Otolaryngology
Massachusetts Eye and Ear Infirmary
243 Charles St., Boston, MA 02114 (USA)
E-Mail christopher_hartnick@meei.harvard.edu

Raol N, Hartnick CJ (eds): Surgery for Pediatric Velopharyngeal Insufficiency.
Adv Otorhinolaryngol. Basel, Karger, 2015, vol 76, pp 7–17 (DOI: 10.1159/000368004)

Nasometry, Videofluoroscopy, and the Speech Pathologist's Evaluation and Treatment

Marie de Stadler · Cheryl Hersh

Department of Speech Language and Swallowing Disorders, Massachusetts General Hospital,
Boston, Mass., USA

Abstract

The speech-language pathologist (SLP) plays an important role in the assessment and management of children with velopharyngeal insufficiency (VPI). The SLP assesses speech sound production and oral nasal resonance and identifies the characteristics of nasal air emission to guide the clinical and surgical management of VPI. Clinical resonance evaluations typically include an oral motor exam, identification of nasal air emission, and analysis of the speech sound repertoire. Additional elements include perceptual assessment of intra-oral air pressure, the degree of hypernasality, and vocal loudness/quality. Clinical speech and resonance evaluations are typically the gold-standard evaluation method until a child reaches 3–4 years of age, when sufficient compliance levels and speech-language abilities allow for participation in instrumental testing. At that time, objective assessment measures are introduced, including nasometry, videofluoroscopy, and/or nasopharyngoscopy. Nasometry is a computer-based tool that quantifies nasal air escape and allows comparison of the score against normative data. Videofluoroscopy is a radiographic tool used to assess the shaping of the velum and closure of the velopharyngeal mechanism during speech production. Evaluation findings guide decision making regarding surgical candidacy and/or the therapeutic management of VPI. Surgery should always be pursued first when an anatomic deficit prevents velopharyngeal closure. Therapy should always be pursued in children who present with velopharyngeal mislearning and/or motor planning issues resulting in VPI. It is not uncommon for children to receive a combination of surgical intervention and speech resonance therapy during their VPI management course. Collaborative decision making between the otorhinolaryngologist and the SLP provides optimal patient care. © 2015 S. Karger AG, Basel

Introduction

The role of the speech-language pathologist (SLP) in the management of pediatric velopharyngeal insufficiency (VPI) is a continuously changing role and one that is based on the evolution of a child's clinical presentation and therapeutic needs. One of the earliest functions of SLP involvement with children with cleft palate and/or craniofacial anomalies is initiation of speech-language therapy as early as at 9 months of age to promote the development of early speech and language skills. It is well documented in the literature that children with a history of cleft palate are at risk for delayed expressive language development [1]. The risk of language delay stems from a variety of potential factors, including frequent ear infections, psychosocial challenges, lengthy or repeated hospitalizations, cognitive deficits, and/or impaired speech production abilities in the setting of the cleft [1, 2]. Children with a syndromic diagnosis are at a higher risk of language delay than children with an isolated cleft lip and/or palate [2, 3]. The focus of speech-language therapy for children under the age of three is typically centered around language stimulation and the quantity of early speech and language skills acquired [4]. Clinical speech and resonance evaluations are utilized during this time to track a child's speech sound repertoire and monitor oral nasal resonance.

Figure 1a is a visual representation of the components of VPI assessment and management when a child reaches 3–4 years of age. At this time, sufficient compliance levels and speech-language skills allow for participation in more structured testing. Instrumental assessment methods are then introduced, including nasometry, videofluoroscopy, and nasopharyngoscopy, to objectively assess velopharyngeal closure and nasal airflow rates. These methods, in conjunction with clinical speech and resonance evaluation findings, are used to determine whether the next step in treatment planning includes surgical intervention and/or speech resonance therapy intervention. Whether surgery or therapy is pursued, the components of the model depicted apply to several different scenarios, including the determination of baseline speech and resonance performance, the evaluation of treatment versus surgical candidacy, and the assessment of post-operative progress. The child may cycle through this model at different phases throughout the course of his or her VPI management. The otorhinolaryngologist (ORL) and SLP collaborate at many points in order to best inform clinical decision making. The best patient care is provided when patients are matched with appropriate clinical treatment courses. Surgery is the gold-standard intervention for children whose speech and resonance profile is the result of physiological limitations of the velopharyngeal mechanism. Speech resonance therapy intervention is the primary avenue of management when the etiology of VPI is related to oral motor planning issues and/or phoneme-specific nasal air emission (PSNAE). Speech resonance therapy should also be pursued as a component of care when the child is stimulable for modifications in speech and resonance using therapeutic techniques. The videos available throughout the chapter allow the reader to explore different assessment and therapy techniques, including the use of instrumental and clinical methods.

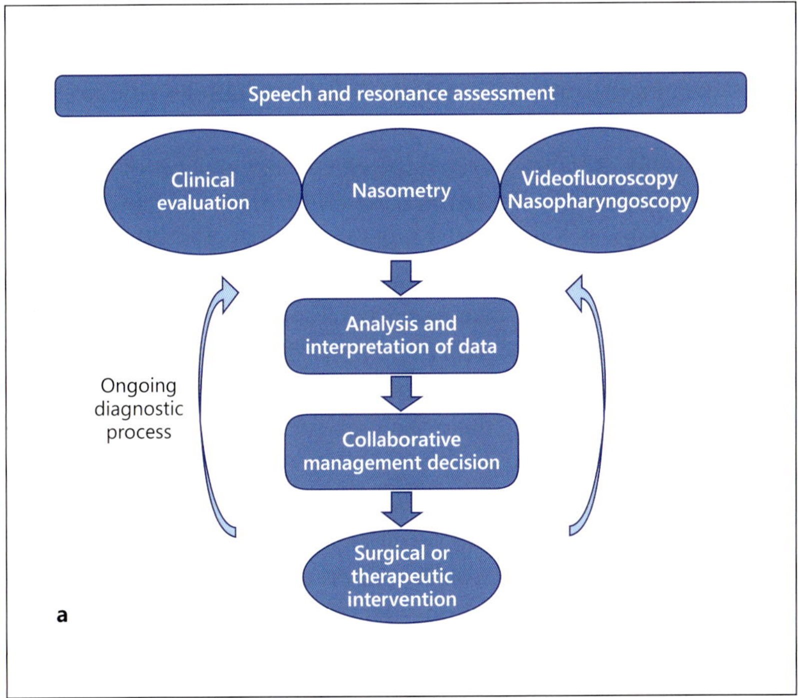

Fig. 1. Speech and resonance assessment when a child exhibits sufficient compliance levels and speech-language abilities allow for participation in instrumental testing.

(For figure 1b, c see page 12.)

Assessment

Clinical speech and resonance evaluations typically include an oral motor exam; identification of nasal air emissions and/or turbulence; and perceptual assessment of vocal loudness, vocal quality, intra-oral air pressure, and the degree of hypernasality perceived [5, 6]. A speech sound inventory is also collected during clinical evaluation to assess speech development and identify whether speech errors are developmental in nature or structurally based in the setting of the cleft or velopharyngeal anomaly. Developmentally appropriate speech errors should not be viewed as concerning when within the normal expected age range for a child. Obligatory errors are the result of anatomical or dental limitations, whereas compensatory speech errors are the result of velopharyngeal mislearning and/or oral motor planning difficulties. Atypical speech errors and compensatory misarticulations are eligible for remediation. Clinical speech and resonance evaluations typically serve as the primary means of assessment for the child under 3–4 years of age due to limitations in compliance and developmental speech-language expectations.

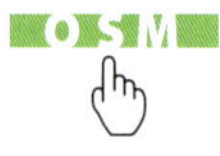

http://www.karger.com/Article/FullText/368004) depicts use of a facilitating /t/ phoneme produced orally to promote oral production of /s/. Auditory feedback is provided with use of a straw and clinician modeling, while visual feedback is provided via a mirror.

Pearls and Pitfalls

The speech and resonance evaluation performed by the SLP yields critical information for appropriate recommendations in the management of VPI.

- Speech and resonance evaluations yield objective and perceptual data with use of the following assessment measures: clinical evaluation (oral motor exam, nasal mirror exam, speech sound inventory), nasometry, and videofluoroscopy and/or nasopharyngoscopy.
- If VPI is related to anatomical limitations of the velopharyngeal mechanism, surgery is pursued first to restore anatomy prior to considering therapeutic intervention.
- If the child presents with functional VPI (e.g. PSNAE), then speech and resonance therapy is the appropriate management avenue, given normal velopharyngeal functioning, for the child's remaining phonemic sound repertoire.
- If oral motor planning difficulties or apraxia is identified as the primary etiology of VPI, initiation of speech and resonance therapy is indicated. A lengthy treatment course should be considered, as characteristics of VPI often resolve when a child's speech precision and oral motor planning abilities improve.
- If VPI is related to both anatomical and oral motor planning difficulties (e.g. a genetic syndrome), collaboration between the SLP and the ORL teams is essential in determining the best sequence of surgical and therapeutic management.
- Assessment and management are ongoing diagnostic processes. The child may receive a combination of surgical and therapeutic intervention throughout the course of his or her VPI treatment.
- A collaborative approach between the SLP and the ORL promotes best-practice decisions, which are beneficial to optimal patient outcomes.

Acknowledgment

There is no potential conflict of interest, real or perceived, for any authors.

Financial Disclosure

None for all authors.
No sources of support, including pharmaceutical or industry.

References

1 Neiman GS, Savage HE: Development of infants and toddlers with clefts from birth to three years of age. Cleft Palate Craniofac J 1997;34:218–225.

2 Hardin-Jones M, Chapman KL: Cognitive and language issues associated with cleft lip and palate. Semin Speech Lang 2011;32:127–140.

3 Hardin-Jones MA, Jones DL: Speech production of preschoolers with cleft palate. Cleft Palate Craniofac J 2005;42:7–13.

4 Kummer AW: Speech therapy for errors secondary to cleft palate and velopharyngeal dysfunction. Semin Speech Lang 2011;32:191–198.

5 Kuehn DP, Moller KT: Speech and language issues in the cleft palate population: the state of the art. Cleft Palate-Cran J 2000;37:348.

6 Rudnick EF, Sie KC: Velopharyngeal insufficiency: current concepts in diagnosis and management. Curr Opin Otolaryngol Head Neck Surg 2008;16:530–535.

7 Kummer A: Cleft Palate and Craniofacial Anomalies: Effects on Speech and Resonance. San Diego, Cengage Learning, ed 2, 2007.

8 Dworkin JP, Marunick MT, Krouse JH: Velopharyngeal dysfunction: speech characteristics, variable etiologies, evaluation techniques, and differential treatments. Lang Speech Hear Serv Sch 2004;35:333–352.

9 Peterson-Falzone S, Trost-Cardamone J, Karnell M: Articulation therapy for school-age children; The Clinician's Guide to Treating Cleft Palate Speech. St. Louis, Mosby, 2005, pp 124–160.

10 Kummer AW, Curtis C, Wiggs M, et al: Comparison of velopharyngeal gap size in patients with hypernasality, hypernasality and nasal emission, or nasal turbulence (rustle) as the primary speech characteristic. Cleft Palate Craniofac J 1992;29:152–156.

11 Kummer AW, Briggs M, Lee L: The relationship between the characteristics of speech and velopharyngeal gap size. Cleft Palate Craniofac J 2003;40:590–596.

12 McWilliams B, Phillips B, Peak BW: Velopharyngeal incompetence; Audio Seminars in Speech Pathology. Philadelphia, W.B. Saunders, 1979.

13 Kummer A: Cleft Palate and Craniofacial Anomalies: The Effects on Speech and Resonance. San Diego, Cengage Learning, ed 2, 2007, pp 377–407.

14 MacKay I, Kummer A: Simplified Nasometric Assessment Procedures, The Mackay-Kummer SNAP Test, ed 2. Lincoln, Kay Elemetrics, 1994.

15 Sweeny T, Sell D: Relationship between perceptual ratings of nasality and nasometry in children/adolescents with cleft palate and/or velopharyngeal dysfunction. Int J lang Commun Disord 2007;43:1–18.

16 Golding-Kushner K: Therapy Techniques for Cleft Palate Speech and Related Disorders, ed 1. San Diego, Cengage Learning, 2001.

17 Ashland J, Rozeboom M: Evaluation and management of speech and resonance disorders; in Rogers DJ, Hartnick CJ, Hamdan US (eds): Video Atlas of Cleft Lip and Palate Surgery. San Diego, Plural Publishing, Inc., 2013, pp 247–254.

18 Baylis AL: Is articulation therapy alone helpful? American Cleft Palate-Craniofacial Association's 69th Annual Meeting and Symposia Web Site (accessed April 16, 2013).

19 Ruda JM, Krakovitz P, Rose AS: A review of the evaluation and management of velopharyngeal insufficiency in children. Otolaryngol Clin North Am 2012;45:653–659.

20 The childhood apraxia of speech association of North America: what is childhood apraxia of speech? 2003. http://www.apraxia-kids.org/ (accessed April 1, 2014).

21 American-Speech-Language-Hearing Association: Childhood apraxia of speech. 2013. www.asha.org/public/speech/disorders/childhoodapraxia.htm (accessed April 1, 2014).

22 Kummer A: Resonance disorders and velpharyngeal dysfunction: evaluation and treatment. Cincinnati childrens speech language pathology. http://www.cincinnatichildrens.org/service/s/speech/hcp/lecture-notes/ (accessed March 4, 2014).

23 Lof GL, Ruscello D: Don't blow this therapy session! Perspectives in speech sciences and orofacial. Disorders 2013;23:38–48.

Cheryl Hersh, MA, CCC-SLP
Department of Speech Language and Swallowing Disorders
Massachusetts General Hospital
275 Cambridge Street, 3rd Floor, Boston, MA 02114 (USA)
E-Mail cjhersh@partners.org

Raol N, Hartnick CJ (eds): Surgery for Pediatric Velopharyngeal Insufficiency.
Adv Otorhinolaryngol. Basel, Karger, 2015, vol 76, pp 18–26 (DOI: 10.1159/000368005)

Nasal Endoscopy: New Tools and Technology for Accurate Assessment

Morgan Bliss · Harlan Muntz

University of Utah Hospital, Division of Otolaryngology, Salt Lake City, Utah, USA

Abstract

In this chapter the technique of nasal endoscopy is discussed. Standardized reporting of nasal endoscopy findings is essential in order to allow communication between different surgeons, speech therapists and endoscopists. Representative videos are provided for the normal examination, for coronal and sagittal velopharyngeal closure patterns, as well as for other anatomical variants of interest. Recommendations for tailoring surgical therapy based on the nasopharyngeal closure pattern are given, although the experience of the surgeon is an important factor for success of any surgical procedure for velopharyngeal insufficiency. Limitations and new frontiers of the technique of nasal endoscopy are also outlined. © 2015 S. Karger AG, Basel

Introduction

Nasal endoscopy has been used since the 1960s to generate a two-dimensional view of velopharyngeal closure in pediatric patients. Rigid endoscopy was initially limited due to the large bulb housing of the scope, but the potential for allowing unimpeded physiologic speech patterns while analyzing anatomic structures was appreciated early on. It was described by Pigott in 1969 [1] as a way of advancing beyond 'lip-read[ing] from the shadows upon the wall.' The development of smaller-diameter scopes and the elimination of the bulb housing allowed improved visualization of velopharyngeal closure patterns. Today, 2.4-mm flexible endoscopes allow for dynamic evaluations of the velopharynx during speech. Nasal endoscopy is not appropriate for every patient with hypernasality. A thorough evaluation by a speech pathologist should be performed first, and the experienced speech pathologist will make an appropriate referral to otolaryngology when a patient's hypernasality is refractory to standard speech therapy techniques.

Patient Selection and Purpose of Exam

D'Antonio and others [2] described six reasons for nasal endoscopy in a 1988 review. These hold true today and are outlined below. Perhaps the most common indication for nasal endoscopic evaluation of velopharyngeal function is to differentiate between learned behavioral causes of speech impediment and anatomic causes of speech impediment. Learned behavioral causes should be suspected when a child demonstrates maximal movements of the velopharynx upon the initial endoscopic exam, but muscular movements are diminished when the child becomes fatigued, frustrated, or excited. While the child with anatomic causes of hypernasality becomes a closely followed patient for the surgeon, the child with learned behaviors causing velopharyngeal insufficiency (VPI) may primarily become the patient of the speech pathologist.

A second indication for a nasal endoscopic exam is to plan for surgical treatment, with the goal of improving speech, or to decide whether a child would benefit from a palatal prosthesis. The process of fitting a palatal prosthesis is also enhanced by nasal endoscopy, allowing for real-time adjustments to the design of the prosthesis with immediate visualization of the resulting velopharyngeal closure [2].

Post-operative evaluation following velopharyngeal surgery in the setting of suboptimal results is a fourth indication for nasal endoscopy. Residual hypernasality or symptoms concerning obstructive sleep apnea should be directly evaluated. The fifth reason to perform nasal endoscopy is to determine if the tonsils and adenoids are contributing to VPI. Finkelstein and others [3] expanded on this indication in their 1994 case series on the topic. They found that anterolateral displacement of the posterior tonsillar pillars due to superiorly hypertrophic tonsils changed the vector of palatopharyngeal movement, resulting in VPI in some cases. Shprintzen [4] described 16 out of 20 patients with tonsillar hypertrophy and VPI whose hypernasal speech resolved completely after tonsillectomy alone.

A final reason to perform a nasal endoscopic evaluation in a patient with hypernasality is to evaluate the degree of velopharyngeal competency prior to maxillary advancement surgery [2].

Children who are determined to be appropriate candidates for nasal endoscopy typically tolerate the procedure well. D'Antonio and others [2] retrospectively reviewed a series of 85 patients aged 3 years and older and found that 89% of exams were completed on the first try. They found that the predictive factors for an inability to tolerate the exam were recurrent or recent epistaxis, an extremely deviated nasal septum, or cognitive impairment with severe expressive language and behavior disorders. Typically, children whose level of receptive and expressive language is at least at the developmental level of a 3-year-old child are able to understand and cooperate with the speech pathologist and nasoendoscopist. Low-dose anxiolytics may be considered during nasal endoscopy in selected children who demonstrate poor cooperation due to anxiety. However, the dose should be titrated so that the child is still able to articulate well. In an unpublished review of 65 children treated at Primary Children's Medical Center in Salt Lake City, 11 children were treated with Versed, 2 mg/kg, during nasal endoscopy in order to manage behavior and anxiety. Good cooperation was achieved in 65% of the children who received low-dose Versed, and moderate cooperation was achieved in 18%. Only 18% of the children who initially appeared to have behavioral and anxiety issues were unable to cooperate with nasal endoscopy after receiving a low dose of Versed [Muntz HR, unpublished data]. In this type of patient, radiographic measures such as videofluoroscopy should be considered. There is no need to perform videofluoroscopy in patients who tolerate nasoendoscopy. While some would argue that videofluoroscopy is useful for determining how high to position sphincter pharyngoplasty, studies have found that placing the flaps as high as possible yields the best results [5]. In this way, we are able to avoid unnecessary radiation exposure from videofluoroscopy.

Nasopharyngoscopy: Technique and Standardized Reporting

Once the decision has been made to perform nasal endoscopy, certain techniques will help to obtain maximum yield from the examination. Endoscopy should always be performed with both a speech pathologist and a surgeon in the room. Explaining the procedure to the parents will help to ease their anxiety so that they can encourage their child to cooperate. A child life specialist can help to create an environment of therapeutic play and provide support during the procedure. After explanation of the procedure, the child's nares are anesthetized with topical anesthetic in combination with a vasoconstrictor. The young patient is then placed in the upright seated position on his or her parent's or caregiver's lap. A member of the medical team helps to keep the child's head still while the parent or caregiver holds the arms and legs. After placing the scope through a naris, the velopharynx is brought into view. Ideally, the entire velopharynx should be able to be seen without having to adjust the position of the nasopharyngoscope. Pulsations: Online supplementary video 1 (for all online supplementary material, see http://www.karger.com/Article/FullText/368005). Occasionally, the scope needs to be passed through both nares to see the entire velopharynx because of a septal deviation.

The palate should first be examined to assess the presence of a muscularis uvula or a submucous cleft with a characteristic midline depression. Alternatively, an occult submucous cleft may be seen with a velum that is flat in the horizontal plane. Some post-operative patients may have scarring or an oronasal fistula. The examiner checks for the presence of pulsations in the lateral pharyngeal walls, which indicate medialized carotid arteries. Normal Exam: Online supplementary video 2 (for all online supplementary material, see http://www.karger.com/Article/FullText/368005). The tip of the scope should be held high in the nasopharynx and as close to the midline of the nasopharynx as possible to minimize parallax. The surgeon or speech pathologist then performs video nasoendoscopy while the patient is instructed to recite a stan-

Table 1. Articulatory phonetics of sample phrases

Speech sample	
Pick up a book	bilabial plosives
Take a turtle	voiceless lingual-alveolar plosive
Go get a cookie	voiced velar plosives
Suzy sees the scissors	sibilants
Mamma made some mittens	bilabial nasal
Bobby and Billy play ball	voiced bilabial stop
A school day for Suzy	sibilants
ssssssssss	sustained fricative
pa pa pa pa pa	repeated plosives

Adapted from [16].

dardized speech sample, which includes all sounds that are appropriately articulated in a speaker's native language. Ideally, samples of connected speech should be tested in addition to repeated plosives and sustained fricatives (table 1). Some smaller children will be able to repeat very limited sample sets. Both nasal and non-nasal consonants should be tested. Maximal movement of the velopharynx is typically seen on sustained fricatives, so this is an important part of the exam [6]. The typical exam lasts a median of 80 seconds [7].

Appropriate articulation can change the closure pattern, so during the endoscopy, focus should be placed on those phonemes that can be accurately produced [8]. In the small child with a developing phonemic repertoire, one may be able to get only bilabial plosives with accuracy. If complete closure is seen with those sounds, there is a good chance that the velopharyngeal closure will be adequate once there is accurate articulation of other developing phonemes. This is often seen in the phoneme-specific /s,sh/.

Golding-Kushner Scale

The Golding-Kushner scale was developed in 1997 as a means to establish a uniform language for describing degrees of severity and closure patterns in VPI. It not only is valuable as a research tool but also allows ease of communication among members of the treatment team who are caring for patients with VPI.

Each lateral pharyngeal wall, the posterior pharyngeal wall, and the velum are assessed individually for the degree of movement. An international working group developed a standardized system of reporting the degree of velopharyngeal movement in 1988 in order to streamline communication between surgeons and speech pathologists within and across medical institutions. In order to minimize the effect of distortion which is intrinsic to nasal endoscopy, the degree of movement is reported as a ratio of movement in comparison with the position of the velopharynx at rest instead of as an absolute measurement. All positions are described on a scale from 0 to 1.0 [9].

When the velum is evaluated, 0 is defined as the position of the palate at rest, and 1.0 is defined as the point where the midline of the palate meets the resting posterior pharyngeal wall. The midpoint of the muscularis uvula is identified, and the trajectory of movement toward the posterior pharyngeal wall is visualized. Coronal Closure Pattern: Online supplementary video 3 (for all online supplementary material, see 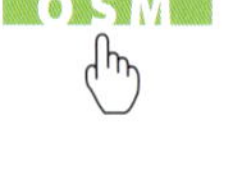 http://www.karger.com/Article/FullText/368005). If there is a submucous cleft or there is no muscularis uvula, the midpoint is defined as the depression in the midline of the palate. If the midpoint only moves halfway to the posterior pharyngeal wall, the score is 0.5. It should be noted whether movement is velopharyngeal or veloadenoidal and whether the uvula occasionally flips into the nasopharygeal port during phonation. If the trajectory of movement toward the posterior pharyngeal wall is asymmetric, this should be noted as well [9].

The degree of movement of each lateral pharyngeal wall is also reported on a scale of 0–1.0. Sagittal Closure Pattern: Online supplementary video 4 (for all online sup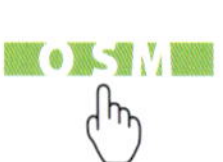plementary material, see http://www.karger.com/Article/FullText/368005). Zero is defined as the position of the lateral pharyngeal wall at rest. If the right lateral pharyngeal wall and the left lateral pharyngeal wall were both to meet at the midline during speech, then each ratio would be reported to have a score of 0.5. If the right lateral pharyngeal wall demonstrated no movement and the left lateral pharyngeal wall touched the right side during phonation, the left wall would be scored as 1.0. The point of maximal lateral motion is used as a reference point to score the degree of movement. If the patient is post-pharyngeal flap surgery, the patient is given a score of 1.0 if the lateral pharyngeal wall touches the lateral aspect of the pharyngeal flap on a given side. Movement away from the midline of the sphincter is given a score of –0.1. The movement of each lateral pharyngeal wall should be described as moving posteromedially, anteromedially, medially, or outward [9].

The movement of the posterior pharyngeal wall is then examined. In 15–20% of the population, Passavant's ridge contributes to posterior pharyngeal wall movement. Passavant's Ridge: Online supplementary video 5 (for all online supplementary material, see http://www.karger.com/Article/FullText/368005). The point of maximal movement of the posterior pharyngeal wall is visualized on a trajectory toward the muscularis uvula or the midline of the velum. If there is no movement of the velum and the posterior pharyngeal wall touches the velum during phonation, a score of 1.0 is given [9]. Significant movement of the posterior pharyngeal wall is rare to see in clinical practice.

The degree of overall closure of the velopharynx is also reported as a ratio on the Golding-Kushner scale. Zero is defined as the size of the gap of the velopharynx at rest during nasal inspiration, and 1.0 is defined as complete closure of the velopharynx, without any bubbling of secretions. A score of 1.0 is given in the case of complete closure, even if there is audible hypernasality. A score of 0.9 is defined as bubbling of secretions through the velopharyngeal port, without any visible gap. The shape of overall closure should be described as either coronal, sagittal, or circular [9]. We have found that describing the degree of the velopharyngeal gap as a percentage is clinically easier to communicate than a ratio and have adopted this method. For example, a completely hypotonic velopharynx would have a 100% gap, and a patient without VPI has a 0% gap.

Tailoring Surgical Treatment

Patients who continue to have hypernasality despite appropriate speech therapy are counseled regarding surgery. We recommend sphincter pharyngoplasty for patients with a coronal or circular closure pattern; a pharyngeal flap for patients with a sagittal closure pattern; and a Furlow palatoplasty for patients with a submucous cleft, longitudinally oriented palatal musculature, and a short palate. A wider pharyngeal flap or sphincter pharyngoplasty is recommended for patients with a larger gap. There are some patients with intermediate closure of both the velum and the lateral pharyngeal walls. Either sphincter pharyngoplasty or pharyngeal flap surgery would be appropriate for these patients. The most important deciding factor in these cases is the experience of the surgeon. Prospective randomized studies have failed to show any significant difference in outcome between sphincter pharyngoplasty and pharyngeal flap surgery [10].

Posterior pharyngeal wall augmentation is used in selected cases in which there is a small velopharyngeal gap that is less than 5 mm.

Palatal lift prosthesis is recommended in rare cases in which patients are poor surgical candidates, for patients who opt to avoid surgery, and for patients who would not be able to tolerate an increased degree of upper-airway obstruction [11]. Palatal Lift Prosthesis: Online supplementary video 6 (for all online supplementary material, see http://www.karger.com/Article/FullText/368005).

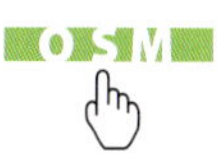

Reliability of Nasopharyngoscopy

A multicenter study was performed in 2008 to the test inter-rater and intra-rater reliability of the Golding-Kushner scale. The nasoendoscopies of 50 patients were reviewed and rated by pediatric otolaryngologists at eight different institutions. The authors found that the scale is more useful in terms of intra-rater reliability than inter-rater reliability. They also found that nasal endoscopy is most reliable for measuring the size of the velopharyngeal gap, somewhat reliable for measuring the degrees of movement and the presence of aberrant pulsations, and less reliable for measuring qualitative features such as notching of the palate. The authors concluded that the scale is not reliable as a tool to be used to compare results across institutions. Intra-rater reliability did not seem to depend on years of experience or the number of patients with VPI evaluated over the past year [7].

Critics of this study have argued that the majority of pediatric otolaryngologists did not perform a high enough volume of endoscopic evaluations of VPI to be considered as experienced nasoendoscopists. This could have affected the validity of the study [6]. Regardless, a standardized teaching tool for using the Golding-Kushner scale has been proposed as a valuable component in order to potentially improve the inter-rater reliability of the Golding-Kushner scale [12].

This standardized teaching tool is published on the American Society of Pediatric Otolaryngology website [12].

Another study by D'Antonio and others [13] collected data from three expert raters and nine novice raters while viewing 95 clinical nasal endoscopic evaluations. This study found that the reliability of expert nasoendoscopists working together is better than the reliability of novice nasoendoscopists.

Use of a computer to capture distances and cross-sectional area measures may improve the accuracy of the exam. If this were done, error calculations would be needed to compensate for the distortions. Though this is certainly possible, one would need to test whether the more accurate assessment actually impacts either research or patient care.

Limitations

Accurate measurement of the velopharynx is limited by distortion of the flexible scope. Pigott has written extensively on the roles of parallax and barreling in the view of the velopharynx obtained with endoscopy. Distortion is still present in rigid nasal endoscopes, but to a lesser degree. Barreling, or the 'fish eye' effect, causes images in the outermost quadrant of the field of view to be one-third the size of objects in the center of the field. Each scope distorts the image to a different degree [14]. Because of this, some have proposed that nasal endoscopy only be used in conjunction with nasopharyngeal fluoroscopic examination. In this era of promoting decreased radiation exposure and medical costs, this is not a feasible option in most practices.

New Technology

New developments in evaluation with endoscopy include flexible endoscopes with a charged coupled device, or 'chip,' located at the distal end of the flexible scope. This new technology has generated excitement among otolaryngologists across all subspecialties. The distal chip eliminates some of the image distortion previously caused by the long flexible wires. However, the 'fish eye' effect is still present in distal-chip scopes due to the nature of the wide-angle lens, which enables a large field of view despite the small diameter of the scope. While there is no published study that has evaluated the diagnostic accuracy of the chip-tip scope for nasal endoscopy, there have been studies in the fields of laryngology and rhinology. One study in the laryngology literature compared endoscopic examination of 34 consecutive patients with rigid endoscopy, high-quality flexible laryngoscopy, and distal-chip laryngoscopy. This study failed to show any additional diagnostic accuracy with the chip-tip scope compared with the high-quality fiberoptic laryngoscope [15].

One emerging niche in endoscopy that may show more benefit in VPI is that of sleep endoscopy. Pre-operative sleep endoscopy in patients who are at high risk for obstructive sleep apnea may help surgeons to decide when to perform a less-aggressive pharyngeal flap surgery or sphincter pharyngoplasty. Post-operative patients with a new diagnosis of obstructive sleep apnea can also be evaluated to determine if multilevel airway obstruction is the cause of sleep apnea or if a simple revision of the velopharyngeal surgery might adequately improve the airway.

Pearls and Pitfalls

- Nasal endoscopy should be used in conjunction with other tests, including auditory speech evaluation, in order to provide a comprehensive understanding of the patient's speech.
- Nasal endoscopy is conducted with the speech pathologist and surgeon in the room at the same time.
- Limitations to endoscopic examination due to patient behavior or copious secretions should be noted.
- The degree of hypernasality should not influence anatomic scoring using the Golding-Kushner scale.

References

1 Pigott RW, Bensen JF, White FD: Nasendoscopy in the diagnosis of velo-pharyngeal incompetence. Plast Reconstr Surg 1969;43:141–147.
2 D'Antonio LL, Muntz HR, Marsh JL, et al: Practical application of flexible fiberoptic nasopharyngoscopy for evaluating velopharyngeal function. Plast Reconstr Surg 1988;82:611–618.
3 Finkelstein Y, Nachmani A, Ophir D: The functional role of the tonsils in speech. Arch Otolaryngol Head Neck Surg 1994;120:846–851.
4 Shprintzen RJ, Sher AE, Croft CB: Hypernasal speech caused by tonsillar hypertrophy. Int J Pediatr Otorhinolaryngol 1987;14:45–56.
5 Riski JE, Ruff GL, Georgiade GS, Barwick WJ: Evaluation of failed sphincter pharyngoplasties. Ann Plast Surg 1992;28:545–553.
6 Shprintzen RJ, Marrinan E: Velopharyngeal insufficiency: diagnosis and management. Curr Opin Otolaryngol Head Neck Surg 2009;17:302–307.
7 Sie KC, Starr JR, Bloom DC, et al: Multicenter inter-rater and intrarater reliability in the endoscopic evaluation of velopharyngeal insufficiency. Arch Otolaryngol Head Neck Surg 2008;134:757–763.
8 Ysunza A, Pamplona C, Toledo E: Change in velopharyngeal valving after speech therapy in cleft palate patients. A videonasopharyngoscopic and multi-view videofluoroscopic study. Int J Pediatr Otorhinolaryngol 1992;24:45–54.
9 Golding-Kushner KJ: Standardization for the reporting of nasopharyngoscopy and multiview videofluoroscopy: a report from an international working group. Cleft Palate J 1990;27:337–347.
10 Abyholm F, D'Anotonio L, Davidson WSL, et al: Pharyngeal flap and sphincterplasty for velopharyngeal insufficiency have equal outcome at 1 year postoperatively: results of a randomized trial. Cleft Palate Craniofac J 2005;42:501–511.

11 Witt PD, Rozelle AA, Marsh JL, et al: Do palatal lift prostheses stimulate velopharyngeal neuromuscular activity? Cleft Palate Craniofac J 1995;32:469–475.

12 Tieu D, Gerber M, Milczuk H, et al: Generation of consensus in the application of a rating scale to nasendoscopic assessment of velopharyngeal function. Arch Otolaryngol Head Neck Surg 2012;138:923–928.

13 D'Antonio LL, Marsh JL, Province MA, Muntz HR, Phillips CJ: Reliability of flexible fiberoptic nasopharyngoscopy for evaluation of velopharyngeal function in a clinical population. Cleft Palate J 1989;26:217–225.

14 Pigott RW: An analysis of the strengths and weaknesses of endoscopic and radiological investigations of velopharyngeal incompetence based on a 20 year experience of simultaneous recording. Brit J Plast Surg 2002;55:32–34.

15 Eller R, Ginsburg M, Lurie D, et al: Flexible laryngoscopy: a comparison of fiber optic and distal chip technologies. Part 1: vocal fold masses. J Voice 2008;22:746–750.

16 MacKay I, Kummer A: Simplified Nasometric Assessment Procedures: The MacKay-Kummer SNAP Test. Lincoln Park, Kay Elemetrics, 1994.

Morgan Bliss, MD
University of Utah Hospital, Division of Otolaryngology
50 North Medical Drive
SOM3C120, Salt Lake City, UT 84132 (USA)
E-Mail morgan.bliss@hsc.utah.edu

Raol N, Hartnick CJ (eds): Surgery for Pediatric Velopharyngeal Insufficiency.
Adv Otorhinolaryngol. Basel, Karger, 2015, vol 76, pp 27–32 (DOI: 10.1159/000368011)

New Technology: Use of Cine MRI for Velopharyngeal Insufficiency

Nikhila Raol[a] · Pallavi Sagar[b] · Katherine Nimkin[b] · Christopher J. Hartnick[a]

[a]Pediatric Otolaryngology and [b]Department of Radiology, Massachusetts General Hospital, Boston, Mass., USA

Abstract

Cine magnetic resonance imaging (MRI) has been used since 1999 to evaluate velopharyngeal function. It allows the visualization of articulatory movement of the velopharyngeal port at rest and during speech. In addition, some studies have shown that it can be synched with audio and can define specific anatomic defects. Cine MRI also provides a non-invasive modality by which velopharyngeal closure can be evaluated. In this chapter, the utility and technique of cine MRI will be described.

© 2015 S. Karger AG, Basel

Introduction

Multiple diagnostic modalities have been used to characterize velopharyngeal insufficiency (VPI). During the speech pathologist's evaluation, perceptual speech analysis, including nasometry, articulation assessment, resonance evaluation, and oral motor function assessment, is essential in diagnosing VPI. However, these tests cannot characterize the pattern of velopharyngeal closure and therefore do not help in determining the ideal surgical (or non-surgical) intervention for treatment. In the otolaryngologist's office, nasal endoscopy/nasopharyngoscopy is used to directly visualize the movement of the velopharyngeal port during specific phonatory tasks (see chapter 3) [1–3]. While this provides excellent information, it only offers a 2-dimensional view at the top of the closure mechanism. In addition, it is invasive and therefore may not be as useful in young children, who may have difficulty performing phonatory tasks while simultaneously tolerating a scope in their nose [3].

Videofluoroscopy is another tool that has been used to evaluate velopharyngeal closure patterns. During this exam, barium is instilled into the patient's nose, and the patient is asked to perform specific phonatory tasks to permit evaluation of the closure mechanism. Three views, specifically, lateral, frontal, and base (also known as the Towne projection) views, are obtained. The height of velopharyngeal closure in relation to the spine and Passavant's ridge is evaluated. A number of limitations have been observed, however, in this type of study. First, the patient is subjected to ionizing radiation, which is always a consideration when performing radiographic studies in children, thus limiting the time to capture images. Second, nasal instillation of barium is irritating and uncomfortable, and the images must be taken at a particular time in relation to administration of the contrast, adding to the difficulty. Lastly, when performed following a surgical procedure, such as pharyngeal flap surgery, this type of study can be difficult to interpret due to the presence of shadows. For all of these reasons, currently, videofluoroscopy is infrequently utilized in the evaluation of VPI [4].

Cine Magnetic Resonance Imaging

Magnetic resonance imaging (MRI) is an appealing option for children since it is a non-ionizing, non-invasive diagnostic modality that can visualize soft tissue in great detail. It was first described in 1999 by Masaki et al. [5] and has become a modality that is being used with increasing frequency for characterizing VPI. In 2002, Kane et al. [6] applied this technology to cleft lip and palate patients, looking at axial views to observe changes in the velopharyngeal port during speech. Recognizing that multiple views were necessary to evaluate the velopharyngeal closure mechanism, Shinagawa et al. [7] reported on the use of cine MRI in the sagittal plane during speech and found that dynamic MRI demonstrated different movement patterns during articulation in a patient with a cleft lip/palate compared with a normal volunteer and provided clear visualization of the velopharyngeal closure pattern.

Taking this a step further, in 2005, Silver et al. [4] published a report on five children who underwent cine MRI with synchronous audio recording at our institution, followed by creation of a movie to evaluate VPI. The authors demonstrated that their method of cine MRI with simultaneous audio was a quick and effective method for the precise depiction of velopharyngeal closure with specific phonatory tasks. It is essential that this type of study be conducted by MRI technicians and radiologists who are familiar with the imaging protocol, as it is currently not widely performed.

Patient Selection

In the senior author's experience, cine MRI is a modality that may be used in essentially all patients who will tolerate the procedure and who have no absolute contraindications to an MRI scan. Children who are claustrophobic, have difficulty executing phonatory tasks on command, have any ferrous implantable objects in their body, or are frightened by the noise of the MRI scanner are not ideal candidates for this modality [4]. Parents are encouraged to remain in the MRI suite with their children to help to comfort their children and maximize compliance.

Cine MRI can be used as an adjunct modality in children in whom nasal endoscopy was not tolerated well or who did not provide enough information. It is also useful for children who have already had surgery but have persistent VPI, as cine MRI can provide greater anatomic detail, with a three-dimensional view as well as dynamic information on the velopharyngeal port, in order to determine the most appropriate next step.

Technique

At our institution, the following MRI imaging protocol is performed. The patients are familiarized with the MRI equipment and asked to practice phonatory tasks in supine position on the table prior to scanning. Children are asked to repeat two standard phrases used by speech pathologists in evaluating VPI. These include 'pick up the puppy' and 'Suzie sees the horse'. The parent or guardian is encouraged to be present in the MRI suite to put the patient at ease. The patient is positioned supine, head first, on the table. In the case of using synchronized audio recording, an MRI-compatible optical microphone is mounted on the head and neck coil, close to the patient's mouth. The microphone is covered by a sound baffle made of foam to enhance sound absorption and decrease the effect of background noise from the scanner itself.

The MRI protocol includes both static and cine sequences. For improved visualization of the upper airway and the levator veli palatini sling, a single acquisition of a sagittal T2-weighted isotropic 3D SPACE sequence is used for the static sequence. From this data set, multiplanar reconstructions in the axial, coronal, and coronal oblique planes are created. These static images are used to evaluate the upper-airway anatomy, tonsillar tissue hypertrophy, and the integrity of the levator veli palatini muscle.

A single-slice 2D FLASH sequence is used for dynamic imaging of the velopharyngeal port, with rapid cine acquisition during phonation. Slice selection is done in three planes, including midline sagittal; axial, at the level of the soft palate at the height of maximal velopharyngeal closure; and coronal, at the center of the oropharyngeal lumen. The imaging time for each cine sequence is 25 s, generating 50 images at a frame rate of 2 images per second. The average time to complete the MRI examination ranges from 25 to 30 min (fig. 1–3).

Limitations

Although cine MRI is a useful modality in which there is significant potential for growth, there are several limitations to the examination. First, the technique by which images are obtained and viewed in a movie format creates room for error due

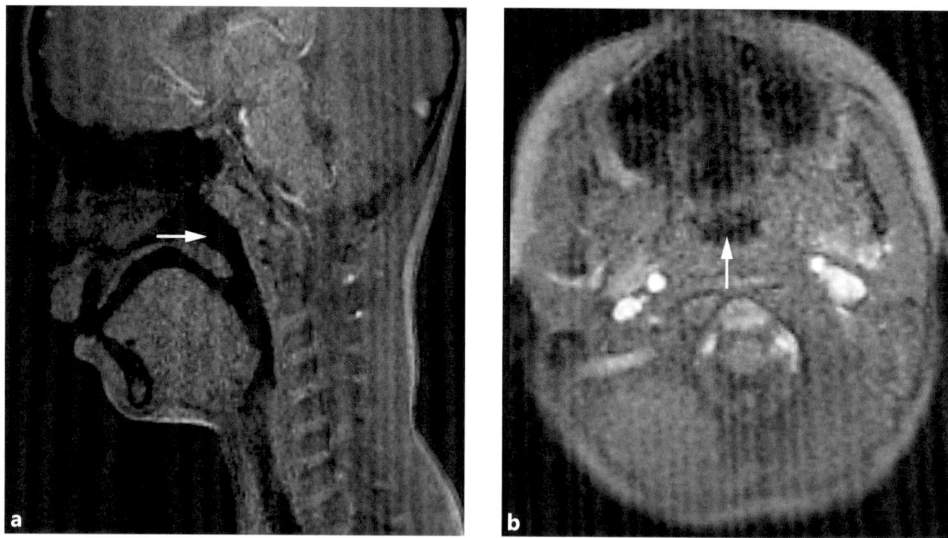

Fig. 1. Cine MRI, 9-year-old with submucosal cleft palate. **a** Sagittal view demonstrating foreshort-ened palate. **b** Axial view demonstrating moderate central velopharyngeal gap.

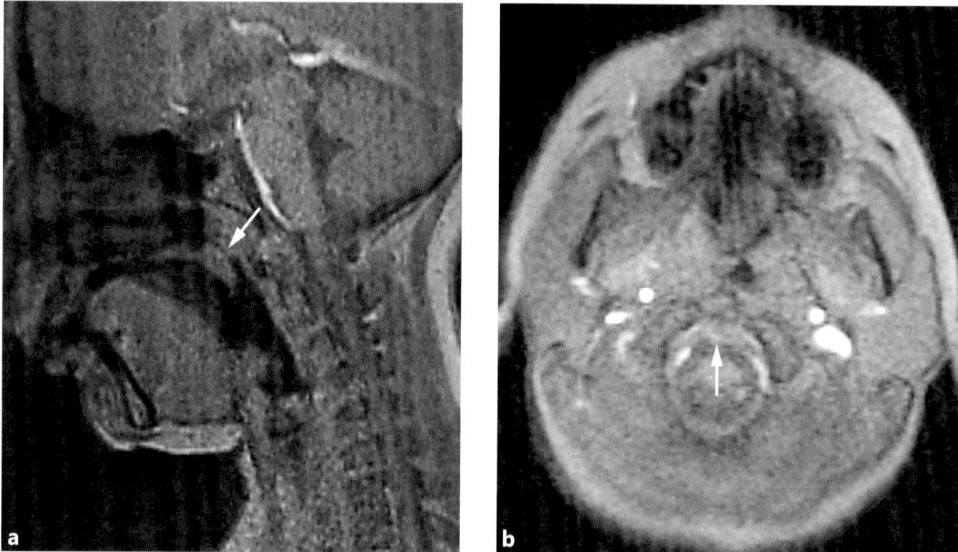

Fig. 2. Cine MRI, 10-year-old with Turner syndrome and VPI. **a** Sagittal view demonstrating touch closure. **b** Axial view demonstrating small velopharyngeal gap.

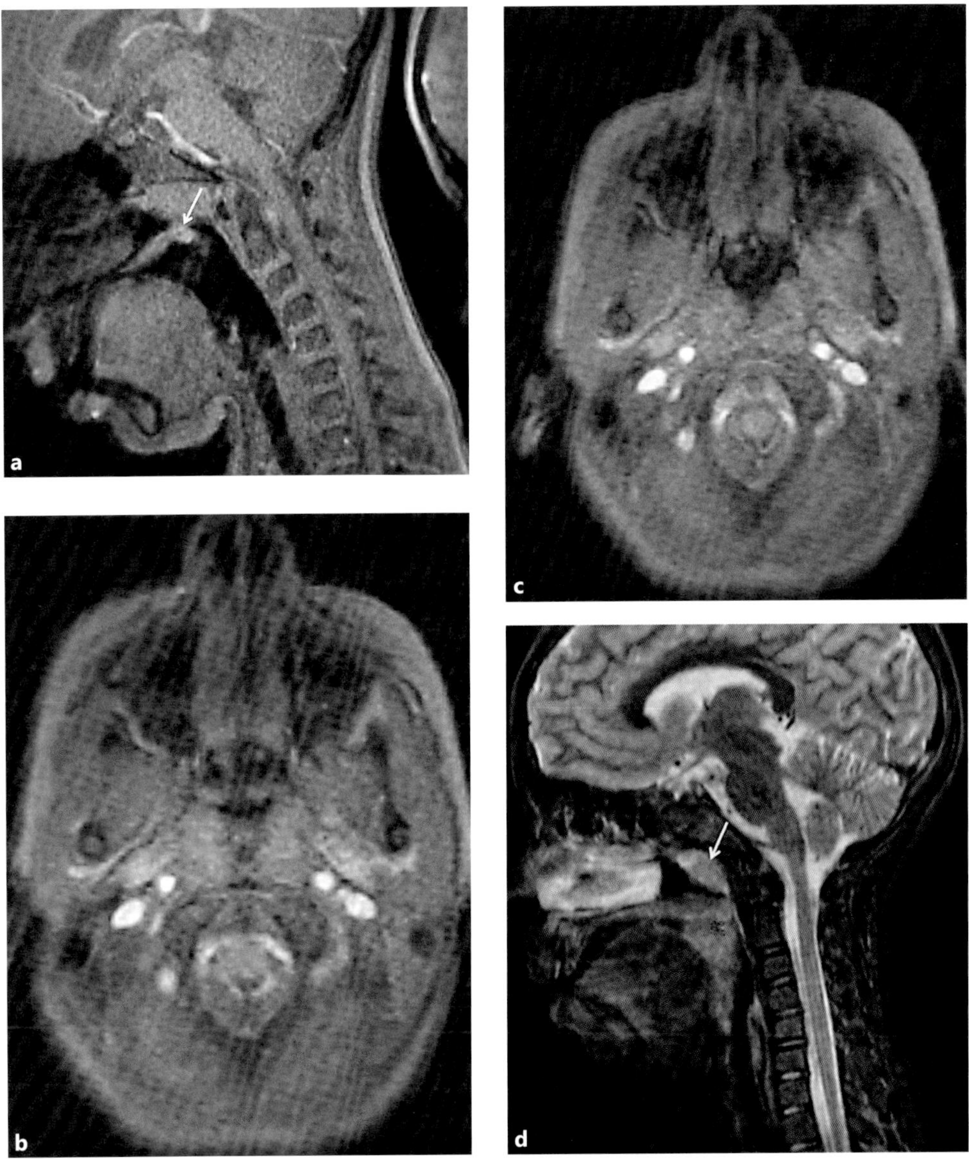

Fig. 3. Cine MRI. **a** Sagittal view demonstrating touch closure. **b** Axial view demonstrating small gap. **c** Axial view demonstrating complete closure in same patient. This indicates that the patient has intermittent VPI. **d** Sagittal view demonstrating enlarged tonsils (red asterisk) and adenoids (white arrow) as possible etiology of VPI.

to the degree of interpolation needed between cine MRI images. It is possible to miss touch closure and therefore acquire false-positive results [4]. This is due to the current technical limitations of MRI, such that cine imaging with diagnostic-quality images can only be performed at lower frame rates compared with a moving picture. Furthermore, the success of the examination depends on the patient's level of

VPI impacts speech, swallowing, and many psychosocial aspects of life in a way that is different from other conditions. Quality-of-life (QOL) instruments provide a method of measuring the value that patients place on their health-related experiences. The challenge is to utilize validated tools to measure these effects. Such tools will help us to understand the impact of the condition and to quantify the clinical improvement that we seek with treatment.

General QOL instruments infrequently contain enough content to fully reveal the impact that the condition has on patients. Condition-specific QOL instruments, in contrast, are tailored to measure how a condition affects QOL and are better able to detect change in QOL than generic instruments are [3]. With this in mind, the ideal patient-reported outcome instrument would be designed specifically for VPI. Such a measure would be useful for (1) helping to inform patient assessment, (2) providing a framework for communicating the impact that VPI has on the patient and the patient's family, and (3) allowing the collection of quantitative data for use in research to improve the care that we provide to our patients.

Patient-Reported Instrument Assessment

Several patient-reported instruments have been used in the VPI population, each with a different type and level of assessment. To help to understand the results and before it is widely used, an instrument should be comprehensively tested to better understand how it functions. The main categories of instrument assessment include validation, reliability testing, and responsiveness. Validation testing, in general, assesses the extent to which the instrument is measuring what it purports to measure [4]. The reliability of an instrument is the degree to which repeated iterations yields the same result [3] and is of importance when an instrument is going to be used before and after an intervention.

Responsiveness, sometimes referred to as longitudinal construct validity, is an instrument's ability to detect a meaningful within-person change in the patient's underlying health status [3]. When a disorder has a treatment of known efficacy, responsiveness is the ability of an instrument to detect change after the treatment [5]. An instrument's responsiveness is assessed in addition to reliability and validity because instruments can be valid but unable to detect clinically important changes [6]. One of the aims of most VPI instruments is their utilization in longitudinal studies evaluating velopharyngeal reconstruction techniques. For this purpose, the instrument should be reliable and responsive [7].

Minimal clinically important difference (MCID) analysis is a method of determining the change in QOL that reaches clinical importance and is often part of responsiveness testing [8]. More specifically, MCID analysis seeks to identify the smallest change in QOL that patients find beneficial. This helps users to understand the clinical implications of a measured change in QOL, both in practice and in research [9]. This analysis is in contrast to tests of statistical significance, which may or may not be clinically important. For example, a large study may find that Treatment A improves a QOL score by 2 points on a 100-point scale compared with Treatment B, with p < 0.05. While this difference may be statistically significant, its clinical importance is not measured by a statistical test.

Effect size reflects the magnitude of change that an instrument measures or a treatment provides. It can be used to assess instrument performance and to compare different instruments' ability to measure change after a treatment of known efficacy. Effect size is calculated using the change in the instrument score with treatment and the standard deviation [10]. An effect size of 0.2–0.5 is typically considered small but clinically important, 0.5–0.8 is considered medium, and greater than 0.8 is considered large [9]. Accumulating information from these various components of comprehensive instrument assessment helps users to understand how the patient-reported instrument functions.

Pediatric Voice Outcomes Survey

The Pediatric Voice Outcomes Survey (PVOS) is a four-question instrument (fig. 1) that was modified from the adult version and validated in a general pediatric otolaryngology patient population. This instrument can be referred to as a functional status instrument in that it measures a patient's perceived speech function. The PVOS was found to be internally consistent (Cronbach's alpha = 0.86) and adequately reliable (intraclass correlation coefficient r = 0.62) [11, 12]. Validation included factor analysis demonstrating construct validity and correlation with a pediatric voice-specific QOL instrument, supporting concurrent validity [13].

During validation of another instrument, the PVOS was confirmed to have adequate test-retest reliability in the pediatric VPI population and to correlate well with a VPI-specific QOL instrument [14]. Further validation of this functional status measure specifically in the VPI population is limited. The PVOS was used in two studies of subjects with VPI and was found to be responsive to changes in speech function after surgical treatment [14, 15].

The instrument's strength of brevity is also its weakness. It has the advantage of a low patient time burden, with four items, but does not have content to measure many of the ways that patients are affected by VPI.

VPI Effects on Life Outcomes

The VPI Effects on Life Outcomes (VELO) survey is a VPI-specific QOL instrument (fig. 2) that has undergone rigorous assessment. Its content was developed from focus groups to help to ensure that it captures the way that patients are affected by VPI [11]. This process helps to provide an instrument with content validity (ensuring that the instrument's domains reflect all of the domains relevant to the condition) [3]. The

The following is a reproduction of a questionnaire form:

Pediatric Voice Outcomes Survey

1. In general, how would you say your child's speaking voice is?
   - ☐ Excellent
   - ☐ Good
   - ☐ Adequate
   - ☐ Poor or inadequate
   - ☐ My child has no voice

The following items ask about activities that your child might do in a given day.

2. To what extent does your child's voice limit his or her ability to be understood in a noisy area?
   - ☐ Limited a lot
   - ☐ Limited a little
   - ☐ Not limited at all

3. During the past 2 weeks, to what extent has your child's voice interfered with his or her normal social activities or with his or her school?
   - ☐ Not at all
   - ☐ Slightly
   - ☐ Moderately
   - ☐ Quite a bit
   - ☐ Extremely

4. Do you find your child 'straining' when he or she speaks because of his or her voice problem?
   - ☐ Not at all
   - ☐ Slightly
   - ☐ Moderately
   - ☐ Quite a bit
   - ☐ Extremely

Fig. 1. Pediatric Voice Outcomes Survey (PVOS).

instrument was modified from its initial length (48 items) to reduce patient burden [11].

The VELO includes a 26-item parent version (VELO-P) and a 23-item youth version (VELO-Y, completed by children 8+ years old). All parents report their perception of their child's QOL, and children over 8 years old self-report their QOL. The items are divided into six subscales, including Speech Problems, Swallowing Problems, Situational Difficulty, Perception by Others, Emotional Impact, and Caregiver Impact (VELO-P only). The total score and subscale score range from 0 to 100, with 100 representing the highest QOL. The subscale scores can be helpful in understanding the nuances of the impact that VPI has on children.

The VELO-P and VELO-Y were found to be internally consistent (Cronbach's alpha = 0.92–0.93) and reliable via test-retest reliability (intraclass correlation coefficient r = 0.85, p < 0.001). The VELO subscales showed similar stability over a time when no change was anticipated [14].

The prospective validation study included all comers with VPI, including newly diagnosed VPI (typically younger children) as well as residual VPI after surgery (typi-

In the past **four weeks**, how much of a **problem** has your child had with (circle one for each question):

Speech Limitations (problems with…)	Never	Almost Never	Sometimes	Often	Almost Always
1. Air comes out of his or her nose when talking	0	1	2	3	4
2. Runs out of breath when talking	0	1	2	3	4
3. Difficulty speaking in long sentences	0	1	2	3	4
4. Speech is too weak	0	1	2	3	4
5. Difficulty being understood when in a hurry	0	1	2	3	4
6. Speech gets worse toward the end of the day	0	1	2	3	4
7. Speech sounds different than that of other kids	0	1	2	3	4
Swallowing Problems (problems with…)					
8. Liquids come from the nose while drinking	0	1	2	3	4
9. Solid food comes from the nose while eating	0	1	2	3	4
10. Others make fun of my child when food or liquids escape through the nose	0	1	2	3	4
Situational Difficulty (problems with…)					
11. Speech is difficult for strangers to understand	0	1	2	3	4
12. Speech is difficult for friends to understand	0	1	2	3	4
13. Speech is difficult for family to understand	0	1	2	3	4
14. Difficulty being understood when not speaking face to face, e.g., as in a car	0	1	2	3	4
15. Difficulty being understood on the phone	0	1	2	3	4
Emotional Impact (problems with…)					
16. Teased because of speech	0	1	2	3	4
17. Child gets sad because of speech	0	1	2	3	4
18. Gets frustrated or gives up when he or she is not understood	0	1	2	3	4
19. Is shy or withdrawn because of speech	0	1	2	3	4
Perception by Others (problems with…)					
20. Treated as if he or she is not bright because of speech	0	1	2	3	4
21. Others ignore my child because of his or her speech	0	1	2	3	4
22. Others do not like to talk on the phone with my child because of his or her speech	0	1	2	3	4
23. Family or friends tend to speak for my child	0	1	2	3	4
Caregiver Impact (problems with…)					
24. I am worried or concerned about my child's speech	0	1	2	3	4
25. I find it difficult to understand my child	0	1	2	3	4
26. My child's speech problem slows me down or inconveniences me	0	1	2	3	4

Fig. 2. VPI Effects on Life Outcomes-Parent Version (VELO-P).

cally older children). The study analyzed younger and older children separately to help to understand the differences that may exist between these groups. The instrument was validated against a variety of other measures utilized in the assessment of this patient population. Understanding these results helps to reveal how the VELO functions and what it is measuring in relation to the other methods of patient assessment.

While no gold standard for VPI exists, perceptual speech analysis is the most widely used measure [16]. Criterion validity (correlation with the gold standard) analysis showed that the VELO-P and VPI severity approached each other but were not associated among all subjects (p < 0.10). Interestingly, the VELO-P was associated with VPI severity among subjects younger than 8 years (r = –0.26, p = 0.05) but not among older children [14].

Construct validation involves a process of hypothesis-testing theorized associations [17]. VELO construct validation tested the association between the VELO and (1) a speech intelligibility deficit (a function construct) or (2) a velopharyngeal gap (an anatomic construct). The VELO-P was associated with speech intelligibility among all patients (p = 0.001), and the association was driven largely by younger patients (r = –0.48, p < 0.001). These results, combined with the criterion validation, show that differences may exist between speech analysis ratings in younger and older children. The association of the VELO score with an endoscopic velopharyngeal gap was moderate (p < 0.01) among all subjects, which was driven by older patients (r = –0.49, p = 0.03) [14]. This analysis, when combined with the correlation found in the speech analyses, shows that the VELO is measuring something that may be missed with other methods of assessment and that differences may exist between younger and older subjects.

Concurrent validity tests the correlation of a new QOL instrument with established patient-reported instruments. The VELO had an appropriate correlation with other QOL and functional status measures, as did most subscales [14].

The VELO instrument was tested for change in QOL 3 months and 12 months after VPI surgery (sphincter pharyngoplasty and Furlow palatoplasty). The VELO-P score improved with treatment by approximately 20 points 3 months post-treatment (p < 0.001). The VELO-P subscales improved at 3 months post-treatment (p < 0.005), except for the VELO subscale Perception by Others. The VELO-Y total score was also able to detect improvement 3 months post-treatment (p = 0.02), but the small sample size (n = 5) limited the power of the subscale analyses [14]. At 12 months post-treatment, similar results were found, except that improvement was identified in all VELO subscales.

Using MCID analysis, we sought to determine the smallest change in the VELO score that patients thought was important. Using a variety of methods, the MCID was determined to be between 7 and 15. Patients who reported that their QOL was 'A good deal better' had a mean change in their VELO score of 19–22, while patients reporting that their QOL was 'A great deal better' had a mean change in their VELO score of 25–43. The analysis also helps to provide context when assessing patients as well as for future studies looking at change in VELO assessed QOL.

Effect Size: Comparison of Instruments

The change in PVOS and VELO scores after sphincter pharyngoplasty and Furlow palatoplasty was analyzed for effect size. For the same treatment, the effect size was large for the VELO total score (1.1) and several VELO subscales, while the PVOS score had a medium effect size (0.6). Instruments with a larger effect size are more able to detect change in QOL or functional status. The VELO may be superior to the PVOS when measuring change in QOL with treatments [14].

Administering the Instruments

Providers should evaluate the available instruments and decide which instrument suits their needs for clinical care and/or research. As described above, the PVOS provides a quick assessment of speech-related dysfunction, whereas the VELO provides comprehensive QOL assessment.

The VELO instrument is typically completed by patients over 8 years old with VPI as well as by the primary caregiver. Children under eight often are unable to complete the 23-item self-report on their own. Parents are encouraged to involve their children under 8 years of age when completing the questionnaire. The instrument is organized in a way that it can be completed quickly and with minimal patient burden. The VELO can be helpful for providers and parents to understand the issues that the patients themselves identify. We have found that parents are often unaware of the issues that are bothersome to the patient. The PVOS has been validated and used with parent report only.

The instruments used thus far have been used primarily in written format. Adaptation to an electronic version could be undertaken if the formatting is similar, so that the previous validation is not compromised. In the flow of a busy clinic, there is often a period of downtime for patients and families. Identifying and utilizing this downtime to capture QOL can help to establish a systematic way of collecting QOL assessments. The QOL instrument is often completed during both the initial and the follow-up speech pathology assessments at our institution. Other centers have chosen to mail the questionnaires to families and to have them bring the packet to their visit. The completed QOL instruments are reviewed with the family, and discrepancies between the child's and the parent's perception of difficulties is discussed. This process often highlights troubles that the child is having about which the parent is unaware. Areas of QOL deficit are reviewed with the family.

Reviewing the instrument with the family can help to provide structure when discussing the impact of VPI on a patient. There are also times when the family's perception of QOL deficit does not coincide with the provider's assessment of speech impairment. It is helpful to identify this in the pre-operative setting to establish realistic goals for surgery.

The more consistently QOL is measured, the better providers will be at understanding VPI-specific QOL in their patients. Integrating such instruments into the flow of the clinic also helps to show families the importance that their providers place on QOL.

Pearls

- VPI impacts QOL in a way that is different from other conditions. Other assessments, such as endoscopy and speech assessment, are not able to measure this impact the way that a QOL instrument can.
- The PVOS is a short validated instrument useful for measuring speech-related functional statusThe VELO is a comprehensive VPI-specific QOL instrument that has been validated and thoroughly assessed.
- The VELO may be more able to detect change in QOL than the PVOS.
- In addition to informing patient assessment, the VELO provides a framework for family discussion.
- Children should complete the VELO-Y as able, and children should be included in the process of parent reporting.

References

1 Witt PD, O'Daniel TG, Marsh JL, et al: Surgical management of velopharyngeal dysfunction: outcome analysis of autogenous posterior pharyngeal wall augmentation. Plast Reconstr Surg 1997;99:1287–1296 [discussion 1297].
2 Sie KC, Tampakopoulou DA, Sorom J, et al: Results with Furlow palatoplasty in management of velopharyngeal insufficiency. Plast Reconstr Surg 2001;108:17–25 [discussion 26].
3 Patrick DL, Deyo RA: Generic and disease-specific measures in assessing health status and quality of life. Med Care 1989;27(3 suppl):S217–S232.
4 Lohr KN: Health outcomes methodology symposium: summary and recommendations. Med Care 2000;38(9 suppl):II194–II208.
5 Liang MH: Longitudinal construct validity: establishment of clinical meaning in patient evaluative instruments. Med Care 2000;38(9 suppl):II84–II90.
6 Guyatt GH, Deyo RA, Charlson M, et al: Responsiveness and validity in health status measurement: a clarification. J Clin Epidemiol 1989;42:403–408.
7 Kirshner B, Guyatt G: A methodological framework for assessing health indices. J Chronic Dis 1985;38:27–36.
8 Terwee CB, Bot SD, de Boer MR, et al: Quality criteria were proposed for measurement properties of health status questionnaires. J Clin Epidemiol 2007;60:34–42.
9 Jaeschke R, Singer J, Guyatt GH: Measurement of health status. Ascertaining the minimal clinically important difference. Control Clin Trials 1989;10:407–415.
10 Cohen J: A power primer. Psychol Bull 1992;112:155–159.
11 Skirko JR, Weaver EM, Perkins J, et al: Modification and evaluation of a Velopharyngeal insufficiency quality-of-life instrument. Arch Otolaryngol Head Neck Surg 2012;138:929–935.
12 Boseley ME, Cunningham MJ, Volk MS, et al: Validation of the pediatric voice-related quality-of-life survey. Arch Otolaryngol Head Neck Surg 2006;132:717–720.
13 Hartnick CJ: Validation of a pediatric voice quality-of-life instrument: the pediatric voice outcome survey. Arch Otolaryngol Head Neck Surg 2002;128:919–922.
14 Skirko JR, Weaver EM, Perkins JA, et al: Validity and responsiveness of VELO: a velopharyngeal insufficiency quality of life measure. Otolaryngol Head Neck Surg 2013;149:304–311.
15 Boseley ME, Hartnick CJ: Assessing the outcome of surgery to correct velopharyngeal insufficiency with the pediatric voice outcomes survey. Int J Pediatr Otorhinolaryngol 2004;68:1429–1433.
16 Conley SF, Gosain AK, Marks SM, et al: Identification and assessment of velopharyngeal inadequacy. Am J Otolaryngol 1997;18:38–46.
17 Health outcomes methodology. Med Care 2000;38(9 suppl):II7–II13.

Kathleen C.Y. Sie
OA.9.220 – Otolaryngology-ENT
4800 Sand Point Way NE
Seattle, WA 98105 (USA)
E-Mail kathleen.sie@seattlechildrens.org

Raol N, Hartnick CJ (eds): Surgery for Pediatric Velopharyngeal Insufficiency.
Adv Otorhinolaryngol. Basel, Karger, 2015, vol 76, pp 41–49 (DOI: 10.1159/000368014)

Prosthodontics Rehabilitation in Velopharyngeal Insufficiency

Matthew Jackson

Consultant in Maxillofacial Prosthodontia to Massachusetts Eye and Ear Infirmary, Brigham, Women's Hospital,
Massachusetts General Hospital, Dana Farber Cancer Institute, and Beth Israel Deaconess Medical Center,
Boston, Mass., USA

Abstract

When surgical correction is less than successful or when children are poor candidates for surgery
due to a large gap, a neuromuscular cause of velopharyngeal insufficiency (VPI), a strong gag reflex,
or unfavorable anatomy, prosthetic intervention can result in the elimination of VPI. Surgery is ideal and best suited for long-term results; however, if needed, prosthetic correction can resolve VPI
and is presented here. Indications for obturators, various designs, and clinical pearls when manag-
ing a child with an obturator are discussed. Correction of VPI must always be considered a multidisciplinary approach involving multiple modalities of treatment and specialties.

© 2015 S. Karger AG, Basel

Prosthetic Terminology

Several appliances are employed to correct velopharyngeal insufficiency (VPI), as fol-
lows:

(1) Obturator/speech aid prosthesis

(2) Palatal lift

(3) Combination of all of the above

An obturator prosthesis is designed for static defects of the palate, specifically hard
palate deformities. Alternatively, a speech aid prosthesis is used to restore a soft palate
defect or a dynamic defect in order to separate the oropharynx from the nasopharynx
[1]. When the velum is inadequate and the ratio of the velar length to nasopharyngeal
depth is excessive, the obturator, in combination with the speech aid prosthesis, sub-
stitutes for this tissue deficiency [2, 3].

When establishing the proper position of the prosthesis into the defect, the neuromuscular activity of the lateral and posterior pharyngeal walls can be stimulated. With

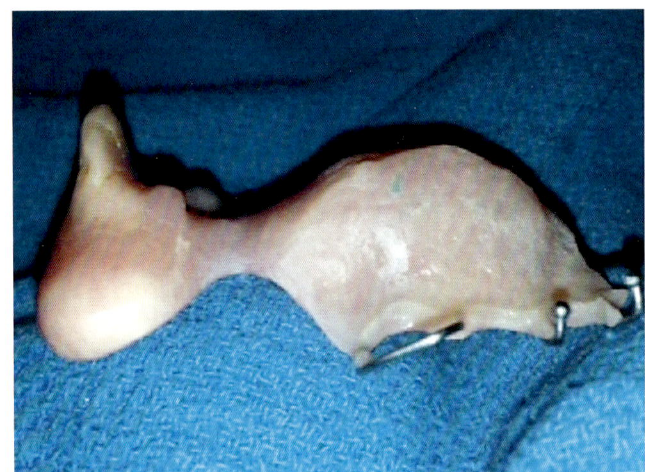

Fig. 1. Meatal obturator extending vertically into the nasal cavity.

time, the pharyngeal musculature strengthens, allowing downsizing of the prosthetic bulb.

Another variant employed for VPI resolution is the meatal obturator or a combination of a meatal and conventionally designed bulb [4]. The meatal obturator itself is static in nature, despite it correcting a dynamic, complex deficiency. Usually, it extends cephalad from the junction of the hard and soft palate in an oblique orientation in order to rest against the turbinates and the superior aspect of the nasal cavity. The disadvantage of this type of prosthesis is that it tends to make the patient's speech hyponasal, which can be altered by creating holes in the prosthesis (fig. 1).

The palatal lift is a prosthesis that is used when the soft palate has proper form and length but the dynamic movement of the soft palate is poor as a consequence of neuromuscular or scarring etiologies. The objective of lifting the palate is to reduce the distance that the soft palate has to traverse in order to produce adequate closure [3–6]. A hybrid of the two previously described prostheses is termed a 'Lift-Obturator' and is useful when the elevation of the velum by itself is still inadequate to develop closure (fig. 2).

Palatal Pharyngeal Landmarks

To construct the dynamic aspect of the prosthesis for the correction of VPI, several landmarks are utilized to objectively improve the positioning of the functional aspect of the obturator/bulb. The three starting landmarks are the anterior tubercle of C1 (Atlas), Passavant's Ridge or Pad, and the horizontal extension of the plane from the superior height of the palatal vault to the pharyngeal walls. Passavant's Ridge is the area of the posterior pharyngeal musculature with the greatest muscle activity and has been found to be the primary pharyngeal structure at the level of the velum. When the soft palate closes, the velopharyngeal port appears as a structure encompassing both

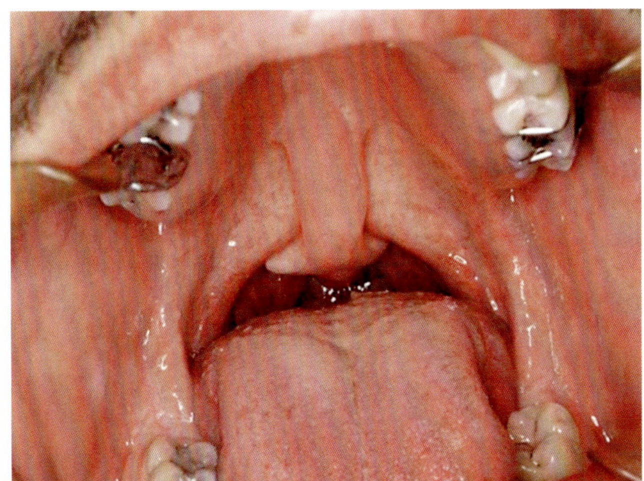

Fig. 2. Palatal lift in place and functioning with closure of the VP portal.

the lateral and posterior pharyngeal walls and is consistently synchronous with velar movement [7]. These landmarks may not meet perfectly, but with the use of functional waxes and help of a speech pathologist, the best possible positioning for speech and swallowing for the patient can be captured in an impression. One must always keep in mind that each segment of tissue may exhibit nonsymmetrical and uncoordinated movement [8].

When dealing with velopharyngeal inadequacy, the pharyngeal bulb/obturator has less active displacement of the tissue compared to the palatal lift, which actively and intentionally displaces tissue of the soft palate and musculature. No matter which specific prosthesis is involved with the correction of VPI, one must remember that the speech compensatory mechanisms for congenital cleft or other oropharyngeal congenital deformities are rooted habits that are not easily eliminated simply by using a palatal prosthesis. A strong multidisciplinary team effort is required to achieve success. On the other hand, a patient with acquired defects has very good speech recovery because they usually present only with hypernasality [9] (fig. 3).

Construction and Fabrication of the Velopharyngeal Insufficiency Prosthesis

The major objectives for a well-fitting prosthesis are support, retention, and stability [10].

Support
Three design features are involved: the occlusal rests, which prevent movement towards the tissue; the major connector, which decreases movement; and the hard and soft tissues, which contact the denture base and underlying tissue.

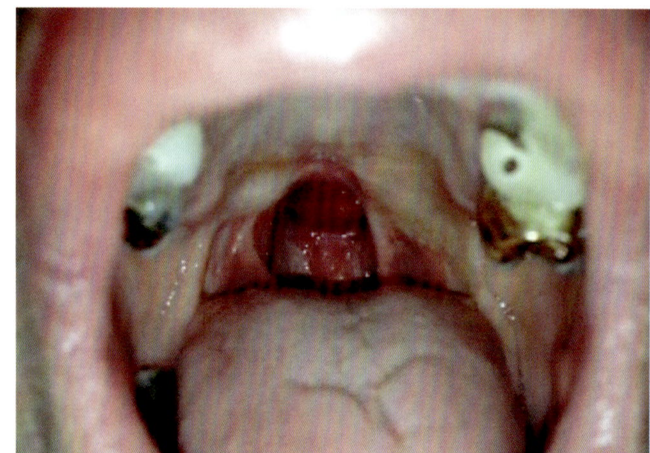

Fig. 3. Resection for a neoplasm of the soft palate. Note the ridge in the midline on the posterior pharyngeal wall, which is Passavant's Ridge.

Retention

The elements involved include the retentive clasps to the undercuts on the primary retainers, which prevent movement and dislodgement; the skin graft within the defect, which creates a retentive interface at the junction of the host and graft; the residual ridges, which provide retention in edentulous individuals; and lastly, endosseous implants, which provide direct retention of the prosthesis. In addition, the occlusal rests prevent rotation and therefore provide indirect retention.

Stability

Stability is provided by designing a minor connector, which prevents lateral movement, as well as denture flanges, which contact the residual ridge and diminish rotation [10–14].

Obturator/Speech Aid Prosthesis

The VPI prosthesis is divided into the oral and pharyngeal sections. The oral component is constructed in the conventional manner, involving all three prosthetic design objectives of maximizing retention, stability, and support. This may involve a partial, complete full denture, an overlay, or any combination of these. Often, malformed and malpositioned teeth have to be removed for proper anatomical form and prosthesis fit.

In general, the procedures include taking preliminary impressions, performing diagnostic articulation for design, using custom trays for final impressions, establishing centric and vertical dimensions, performing registration for articulation, and trying the tentative setup for verification of centric, vertical dimension, aesthetics, and function. If all are verified and if the patient approves, the case goes to completion using the final materials of choice.

Jackson

Often, it is recommended to first insert the oral prosthesis, thus allowing the patient to adjust accordingly. This is especially helpful for a patient with a gag reflex. However, one can simultaneously fabricate the oral and pharyngeal sections together, thus accelerating the reestablishment of speech and swallowing. This is often necessary for the acquired or traumatic defects experienced by the pediatric population.

When constructing the pharyngeal portion, a retentive loop extension is posteriorly fastened to the oral prosthesis into the distally located defect without interfering with the residual soft tissue. The loop will facilitate retention of the impression materials into the pharyngeal defect. A thermoplastic modeling compound is placed around the extension. When heated properly, the modeling compound molds to the pharyngeal deficiency until functional contact occurs. The material can be added or removed at the discretion of the practitioner. With the addition of a modeling compound, the prosthesis is placed back into the mouth, and the patient is instructed to flex his or her neck forward, tucking the chin into the chest, which records the position of the atlas on the compound impression.

Laterally, the bulb is defined by the rotation and flexion of the neck and by having the patient touch his/her left and right shoulders with the side of his/her face. Upon completion, the modeling compound should not permit air or liquids to flow between the oral and nasal cavities. The impression is then removed from the mouth and chilled, which establishes the boundaries of the pharyngeal defect.

Once hardened, 1 mm of the compound is circumferentially removed with a scalpel blade, and mouth flowing functional wax (i.e., Adaptol, Iowa, or Korecta wax) is added. Functional flowing waxes at body temperature mold and define the anatomical contours of the tissues they are impressing. The prosthesis is then reinserted, and the previously performed maneuvers are repeated.

In addition, the patient is asked to swallow and speak, and the functional wax is left in the oral cavity for 10 minutes for each repetitive insertion. Any exposure of the underlying wax revealing the compound is cut back, and additional functional material is added. The impression is then reinserted, and exercises and procedures are again performed. Upon completion, nasal breathing as well as swallowing should be comfortable and unrestricted. If additional space is necessary for nasal breathing, material is removed laterally with the understanding that this may lead to hypernasality. Once the low-fusing functional wax is developed circumferentially and breathing and swallowing are comfortable, the impression is removed and chilled.

In the case where the soft palate is anatomically intact but the length and/or function is inadequate to close the velopharyngeal portal, the obturator must be able to cross comfortably across the soft palate in order to obturate the pharyngeal deficiency. In addition, the prosthesis itself can be a diagnostic tool over time and often indicates the relative success of a pharyngeal flap.

The meatal obturator is mainly indicated when the posterior pharyngeal area elicits a gag reflex despite desensitization of the gag reflex, and the design features are distinct. The meatal 'bulb' extends statically and projects vertically at the posterior or

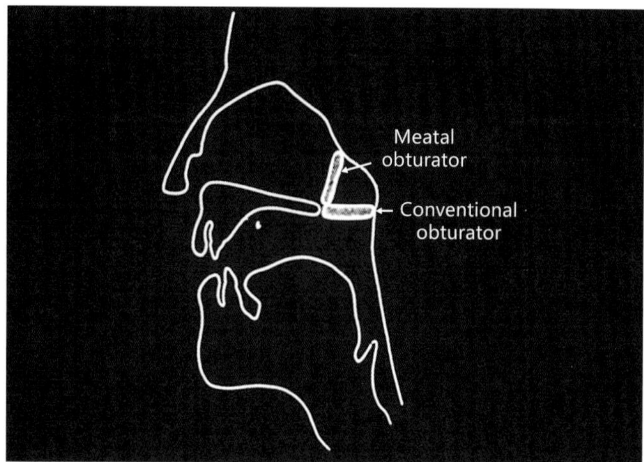

Fig. 4. The two different positions of an obturator.

distal end of the oral prosthesis, usually at the junction of the hard and soft palate (fig. 1, 4) Obturation is obtained against the posterior nasal turbinates and the superior aspect of the nasal cavity (fig. 4).

The obturator itself is closer to the hard palate, resulting in less torque placed on the pharyngeal/oral portion, which decreases dislodgement. The speech after insertion tends to be hyponasal sounding, as if the patient has a cold and has difficulty with nasal breathing. The remainder of the construction is the same as previously mentioned. The full extent of the defect is then obtained by the compound, cut back, and developed with functional wax against the nasal choanae. The prosthesis is then completed in the conventional way, into a definitive prosthesis in acrylic. Once in the mouth and adjusted, properly angulated holes are bored on either side of the meatal vertical extension to improve nasal breathing and hyponasal speech and to limit nasal reflux, which is a shortcoming of this design.

The Palatal Lift Prosthesis

When the soft palate is intact and of proper length but nonfunctional or inadequately functional to close the pharyngeal port, a palatal lift prosthesis can be utilized to mechanically lift the immobile soft palate. Fibrosis may be of major concern and could result from surgeries or from irradiation of the pharyngeal area from childhood neoplasms. Objectively, the soft palate is elevated to the correct superior position, with gravity, elasticity, fibrosis, and muscle activity tending to dislodge the prosthesis. This is resisted by the retention that is established by the oral aspect of the prosthesis, which attaches to the teeth. However, edentulous patients will not develop as much resistance to dislodging forces, and adjunct retention can be obtained with the use of denture adhesives or endosseous implants (fig. 5, 6).

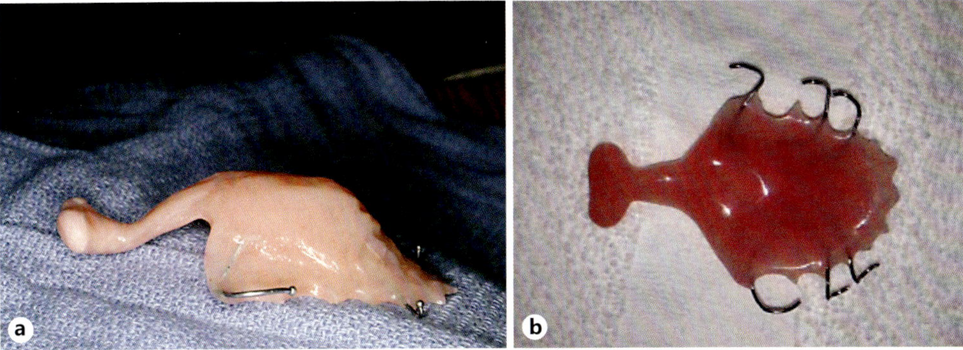

Fig. 5. Horizontal (**a**) and vertical (**b**) views of the completed lift prosthesis. Note the elevation of the distal aspect of the prosthesis placing the soft palate into the proper position for closure of the VP portal (**a**).

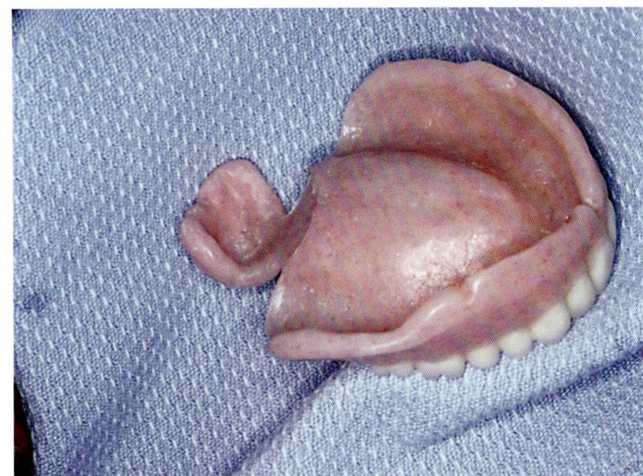

Fig. 6. Edentulous 'Lift-Obturator' prosthesis relying on suction and a peripheral seal as well as dental adhesives for stability and retention.

Again, similar techniques and materials as for the obturator are employed when lifting the soft palate. If nasal breathing becomes a problem, lateral reduction of the lift will improve nasal breathing but may induce some hypernasality. The elevation of a flaccid soft palate will lessen the torque and dislodgement. On the other hand, a scarred, fibrotic, or taut soft palate can make dislodgement more significant and requires optimizing the retention developed from the oral aspect of the prosthesis.

Clinical Pearls: How to Choose the Best Fit for the Right Patient

Deciding which patient would benefit most from a palatal prosthesis can be difficult, as one must consider the etiology of VPI, age of the patient, compliance of the patient, fit of the prosthesis, and cost, among other factors. While a child of any age can be considered a candidate, the attitude and fears of both the child and parents must be addressed. Often the child will not tolerate the required procedures. Furthermore, in cases where he/she does allow it, long-term prosthesis use is often too much for a child. Typically by early adolescence (age 11–12) and beyond, the patient becomes more cooperative and understands the benefit that is received from the prosthesis. In children who have a strong gag reflex, deprogramming the reflex can help improve compliance. This can be done by moving a tongue blade or finger to the back of the throat from the hard palate several times daily within a short period of time. The child and parents have to be vigilant to do these exercises. Often a prosthesis can be added to or subtracted from according to the tolerance of the patient and the need to modify the speech and/or swallowing mechanism. Lastly, infants often tolerate the prosthesis well because they are not aware enough to resist.

In deciding between a palatal lift and an obturator, one should remember that a palatal lift is best when the soft palate is of normal length for closure of the oropharyngeal portal but has inadequate muscle function to elevate the soft palate to close the portal. In addition, if there is a space behind the elevated soft palate after placing a palatal lift, obturation of some sort will be required, whether it is a combination of a lift/obturator, speech bulb, meatal prosthesis or any combination of these.

Finally, the cost of the prosthesis should be discussed with the family when making these choices. While prosthodontists are licensed as dentists, dental codes do not cover these prostheses, as they are deemed to be medically necessary. Therefore, they should be covered as a congenital deformity/pre-existing malady under the new healthcare law. However, this should be confirmed with the individual carrier prior to fashioning the prosthesis to ensure that the patient's family can afford the cost.

In summary, successfully caring for the pediatric population with VPI must be a team effort between the speech pathologist, surgeon, orthodontist, prosthodontist, social workers, and family. However, overall success must include the successful cooperation of the patient because without his/her cooperation and resolve, success cannot be achieved. Dr. Herbert Cooper stated 'A physical defect such as a cleft palate, does not constitute a social handicap'. Although it will be always present, the patient must learn to accept things which cannot be changed, must be encouraged to change things than can be changed, and must be taught to know the difference' [15].

References

1 Yenisey M, Cengiz S, Sarıkaya I: Prosthetic treatment of congenital hard and soft palate defects. Cleft Palate Craniofac J 2012;49:618–621.

2 Moore D, McCord JF: Prosthetic dentistry and the unilateral cleft lip and palate patient. The last 30 years. A review of the prosthodontic literature in respect of treatment options. Eur J Prosthodont Restor Dent 2004;12:70–74.

3 Beumer J, Curtis TA, Marrunick MT: Maxillofacial Rehabilitation: Prosthodontic and Surgical Considerations, ed 1. St. Louis, Medico Dental Media International Inc., 1996.

4 Rahn AO, Boucher LJ: Maxillofacial Prosthetics: Principles and Concepts. Philadelphia, W.B. Saunders Co., 1970.

5 Shifman A, Finkelstein Y, Nachmani A, et al: Speech-aid prostheses for neurogenic velopharyngeal incompetence. J Prosthet Dent 2000;83:99–106.

6 Reisberg DJ: Dental and prosthodontic care for patients with cleft or craniofacial conditions. Cleft Palate Craniofac J 2000;37:534–537.

7 Glaser ER, Sholnick ML, McWilliams BJ, Shprintzen RJ: The dynamics of Passavant's ridge in subjects with and without velopharyngeal insufficiency – a multi-view videofluoroscopic study. Cleft Palate J 1979;16:2–33.

8 Yoshida H, Michi K, Yamashita Y, et al: A comparison of surgical and prosthetic treatment for speech disorders attributable to surgically acquired soft palate defects. J Oral Maxillofac Surg 1993;51:361–365.

9 Plunk DM, Weinberg B, Chalian VA: Evaluation of speech following prosthetic obturation of the surgical acquired defects. J Prosthet Dent 1981;45:627–638.

10 Management of the Soft Palate Defect. np. www.sid.cu/galerias/pdf/sitosis/prothesis/management_management_of_the_soft_palate_defect_steven_eckert.pdf (accessed 3/3/2014).

11 Folkins JW: Velopharyngeal nomenclature: incompetence, inadequacy, insufficiency, and dysfunction. The Cleft Palate Craniofacial Journal. http://digitallibrary.pitt.edu/cleftpalate (accessed 3/10/2014).

12 Tuna SH, Pekkan G, Gumus HO, et al: Prosthetic rehabilitation of velopharyngeal insufficiency: pharyngeal obturator prostheses with different retention mechanisms. Eur J Dent 2010;4:81–87.

13 Rogers DJ, Harnick CJ, Hamdan US: Video Atlas of Cleft Lip and Palate Surgery. San Diego, Plural Publishing, 2013.

14 Zemnick C: The adjustable palatal lift prosthesis. Columbia University and Bronx Veterans Medical Center. www.maxillofacialprosthetics.org/2010Presentation/AAMP (accessed 3/7/2014).

15 Cooper HK, Long RE, Cooper JA, Mazaheri M, Millard RT: Psychological, orthodontic and prosthetic approaches in rehabilitation of the cleft palate patient. Dent Clin North Am 1960;4:383–393.

Dr. Matthew Jackson
Head and Neck Svc, 11th floor
243 Charles St.
Boston, MA 02061 (USA)
E-Mail matthew_jackson@meei.harvard.edu

Raol N, Hartnick CJ (eds): Surgery for Pediatric Velopharyngeal Insufficiency.
Adv Otorhinolaryngol. Basel, Karger, 2015, vol 76, pp 50–57 (DOI: 10.1159/000368016)

Superiorly Based Pharyngeal Flap

Nikhila Raol · Christopher J. Hartnick

Fellow, Pediatric Otolaryngology, Massachusetts Eye and Ear Infirmary, Boston, Mass., USA

Abstract

First described in 1875 by Schoenborn as an inferiorly based flap, the pharyngeal flap is the most common surgical procedure performed for velopharyngeal insufficiency. Having undergone numerous modifications since its conception, the pharyngeal flap is now primarily designed as a superiorly based flap and is most effective for patients with good lateral wall motion but limited anterior-posterior motion due to poor palatal excursion. The primary aims of this chapter are to provide the clinician with indications for when to consider utilizing the superiorly based pharyngeal flap and to give a stepwise description of how to perform the procedure. © 2015 S. Karger AG, Basel

Introduction

The superiorly based pharyngeal flap is the most commonly performed procedure for velopharyngeal insufficiency (VPI), and it is ideal for patients with good lateral pharyngeal wall movement but poor palatal movement, resulting in a central velopharyngeal gap. The goal of this surgery is to utilize myomucosal tissue from the posterior pharynx to bridge this central gap, leaving lateral ports on either side of the flap to prevent complete nasal obstruction resulting in obstructive sleep apnea (OSA) and hyponasality. This technique was first described as an inferiorly based flap by Schoenborn in 1875 [1]; however, he later modified this to a superiorly based flap, as he found that the short length of the inferiorly based flap and its tendency to contract and pull the soft palate downward made it less than ideal. In 1930, Padgett introduced and popularized the use of this flap across America [2]. In the 1970s, Hogan and Shprintzen made additional contributions by describing lateral port control and tailor-made flaps via preoperative videofluoroscopy and nasopharyngoscopy, respectively [3, 4].

The frequent use of this flap can likely be attributed to its high success rates, with Shprintzen reporting up to an 80% success rate when the flap is used randomly in patients with VPI [4]. Sullivan et al. reviewed outcomes of 79 nonsyndromic patients who required pharyngeal flap for VPI following cleft palate repair and found improvement of velopharyngeal function to normal or borderline in 97% of patients, which is comparable to the reported success rates of 78–98% [5–9]. In the senior author's experience, the success rate is about 90–95% with careful selection via appropriate preoperative evaluation using nasopharyngoscopy and videofluoroscopy.

The primary complications of this procedure include complete or partial dehiscence of the flap causing persistent VPI and OSA. Witt et al. demonstrated an approximately 20% revision rate in a review of 65 patients, with dehiscence being the most common reason for revision [10]. The incidence of OSA is about 2–10% following pharyngeal flap; Ysunza et al. noted that nearly all patients (14/15) had resolution of OSA with tonsillectomy. This finding was independent of flap size [11]. Sullivan reported an incidence of approximately 2% as well, despite addressing enlarged tonsils prior to surgery for VPI [5].

Due to the design of the flap, consideration must be given to the location of the internal carotid artery in each individual patient because there are known syndromes, such as 22q11 deletion syndrome, where a medial/retropharyngeal course of the internal carotid artery is not uncommon. At our institution, we have identified additional syndromic patients with medialized carotids, leading to a change in the operative plan. Therefore, vascular imaging is obtained in all patients with 22q11 deletion syndrome and in select patients with other syndromes based on office evaluation. While some report that the use of the pharyngeal flap is safe in patients with medialized carotid arteries, it is considered a relative contraindication by the senior author given the possibility of severe hemorrhage intraoperatively and of devastating outcomes if a wound infection ensues and reaches the carotid region.

Patient Evaluation

1. Office Visit.
a. History, including genetic disorders, previous operations, cleft palate, etc.
b. Physical exam, including nasopharyngoscopy to evaluate the velopharyngeal closure pattern and evidence of medialized carotid arteries (see Chapter 3). A sagittal closure pattern is most ideal for superiorly based pharyngeal flap.
2. Speech pathology evaluation, including fluoroscopy if recommended by a speech pathologist (see Chapter 2).
3. Adjunct studies as needed, including cine MRI (see Chapter 4) and/or vascular imaging.

Indications

- A wide central velopharyngeal gap that is greater than one-third the width of the palate. When the width is one-third or less, posterior pharyngeal wall augmentation can also be considered. When the distance between the soft palate and posterior

pharyngeal wall can be closed with gentle pressure on the soft palate, a palatal lengthening procedure, Furlow palatoplasty, can be considered. When the distance between the soft palate and the posterior pharyngeal wall appears too large and when a flap that is long enough cannot be created, a palatal lift or obturator should be considered.
- Persistent VPI due to a shortened soft palate following primary cleft palate repair.
- Persistent VPI following other unsuccessful procedures.

Contraindications

- Pre-existing OSA. The tonsils should be evaluated for hypertrophy, and if needed, a tonsillectomy should be performed. This is typically performed 6 weeks prior to the primary surgery for VPI, but it has also been described as a simultaneous procedure.
- Midline/medial carotid vasculature (relative).
- Neuromuscular deficits causing an immobile palate or clefts that are too wide to be repaired where an obturator/palatal lift is needed.

Anesthesia Considerations

- Midline endotracheal tube – an Oral Rae or armored tube is preferred to prevent 'kinking' of the tube during the course of the procedure.
- An in-depth discussion with the anesthesiologist should be conducted prior to the start of the procedure. It is imperative to relay the need for an awake extubation due to the newly created obstruction in the nasopharynx. The patient should not be extubated during phase 2 and should be completely awake prior to removing the tube. A tongue stitch should be placed prior to the end of the procedure for retraction in case of obstruction. A laryngeal mask airway should be kept nearby in the event of airway difficulty.

Materials

- Crowe-Davis mouth gag/tonsil set.
- Colorado tip Bovie.
- Multiple 4-0 Vicryl sutures on a small taper needle.
- Two 3-0 uncuffed endotracheal tubes.

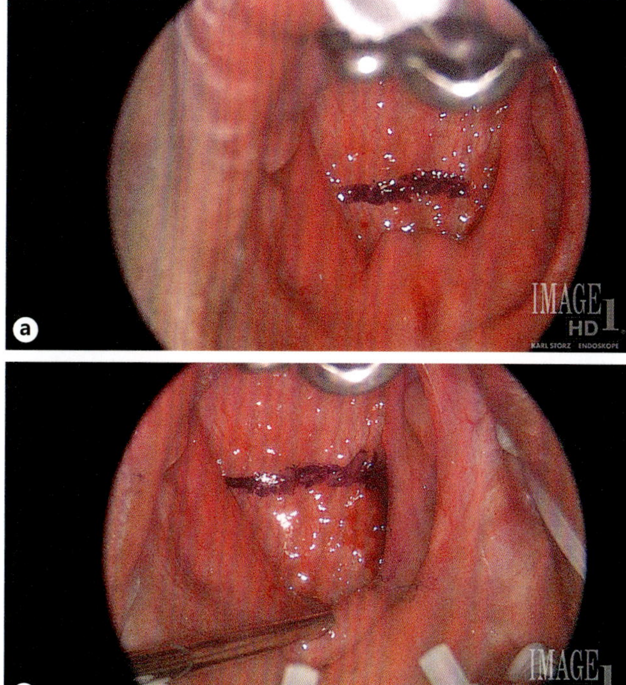

Fig. 1. Marking the inferior aspect of the superiorly based pharyngeal flap with the soft palate in its normal position (**a**) and with the soft palate retracted superiorly (**b**).

Set-Up

- A modified Rose position with generous shoulder roll for neck extension if the surgeon is seated for the procedure.
- Mark the proposed posterior pharyngeal wall incisions with either Gentian Violet or a surgical marker (fig. 1). The lateral borders of the flap are marked at the posterior tonsillar pillars. The surgeon can use a Hurd to measure the approximate distance between the soft palate and the posterior pharyngeal wall (fig. 2). This measurement is then used to approximate the length of the pharyngeal flap.
- Local injection with lidocaine and 1:100,000 epinephrine along the proposed incision lines and the inferior soft palate, with a wait time of 5–7 minutes to ensure adequate hemostasis.

Procedure

Superiorly-Based Pharyngeal Flap: Online supplementary video (for online supplementary material, see http://www.karger.com/Article/FullText/368016).

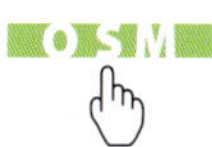

- An incision is made with a Colorado tip Bovie through the mucosa and muscle of the posterior pharyngeal wall, as marked, until the prevertebral fascia is reached (fig. 3).

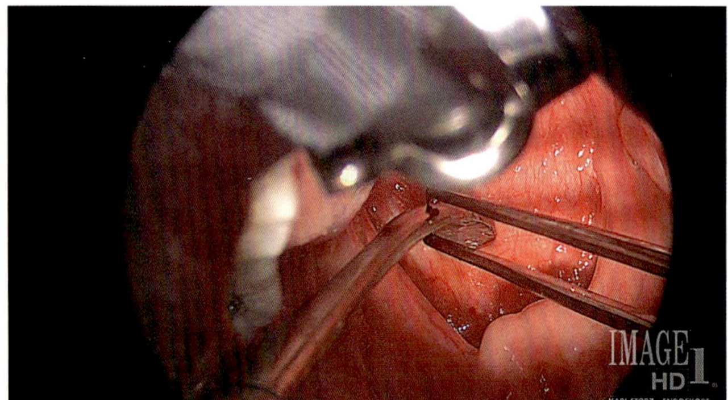

Fig. 2. Measuring the distance from the soft palate to the posterior pharyngeal wall.

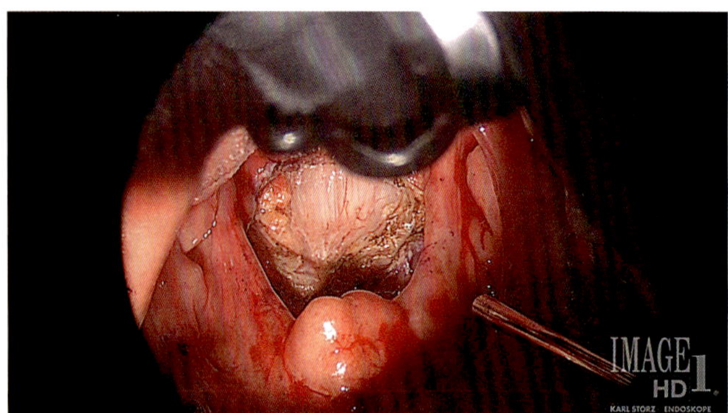

Fig. 3. An incision down to the prevertebral fascia.

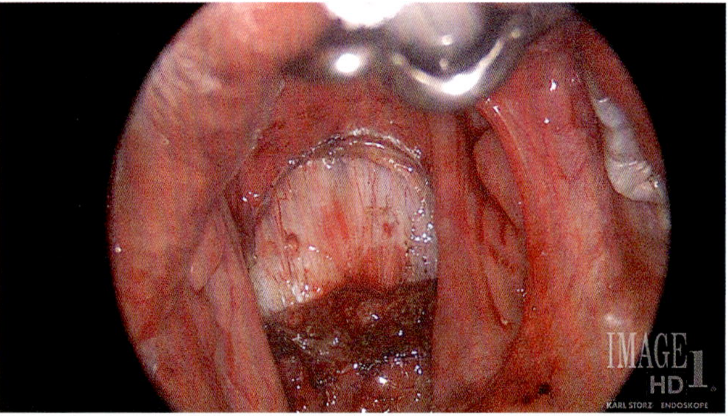

Fig. 4. The flap elevated into the nasopharynx.

- The myomucosal flap is raised in an inferior to superior fashion into the nasopharynx with a Bovie and a peanut, using a pickup with teeth to gently grasp the flap (fig. 4).
- The soft palate is grasped, and the posterior surface of the inferior edge is demucosalized using the Colorado tip Bovie until the muscle is visible.

Raol · Hartnick

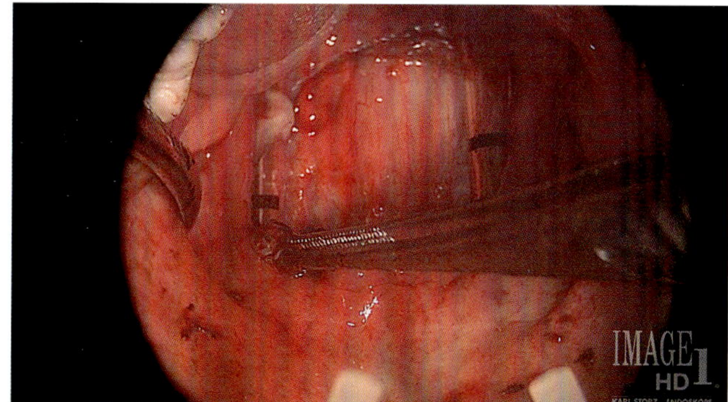

Fig. 5. 3-0 endotracheal tubes in place to estimate the lateral ports.

- Two 3-0 uncuffed endotracheal tubes are then passed through the nose, one through each nostril, until each is pulled into the oropharynx along the lateral edges. These are used to create the lateral ports (fig. 5).
- A 4-0 Vicryl suture is then used to inset the pharyngeal flap into the soft palate. Care must be taken to take thick bites that contain muscle from the flap and to suture this tissue to the muscle and mucosa of the soft palate.
- The lateral edges of the flap should be inset first, with the endotracheal tubes placed on the outside of the suture. A total of four sutures (two lateral, two central) is typically adequate (fig. 6).
- The endotracheal tubes are withdrawn through the nose.
- A dental mirror is used to examine the lateral ports. If they appear to be too large, additional Vicryl sutures may be placed.
- The posterior pharyngeal wall is closed with Vicryl sutures using 2–3 simple interrupted stitches. Care should be taken to avoid bunching.
- A 2-0 silk suture is then placed through the tongue as a retraction suture in case obstruction occurs postoperatively. This suture is taped to the cheek (fig. 7).
- The mouth gag is then carefully removed, and the patient is turned over to anesthesia for awake extubation.

Postoperative Care

- The patient should be monitored in an intensive care unit setting overnight for OSA.
- Care must be taken to prevent trauma to the repair. This might involve use of arm restraints during the postoperative period if the child has a propensity to put his/her fingers in the mouth. Additionally, the use of 'sippy' cups and straws should be avoided for approximately 3 weeks after surgery.
- Solid foods should be of a pureed consistency for 3 weeks following surgery. Foods such as breadcrumbs or crackers should be avoided to keep particles from getting trapped in the posterior pharyngeal wall.

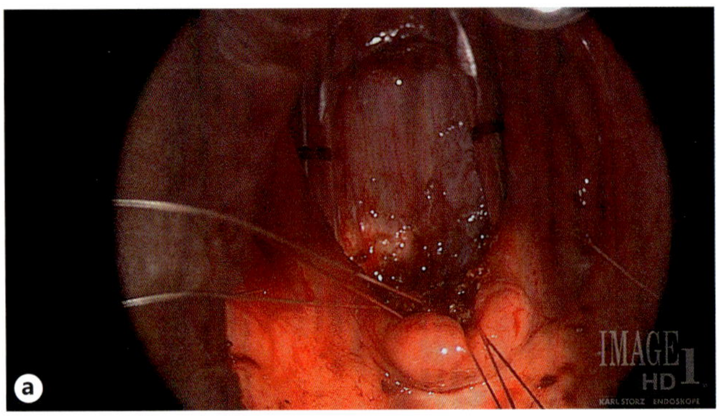

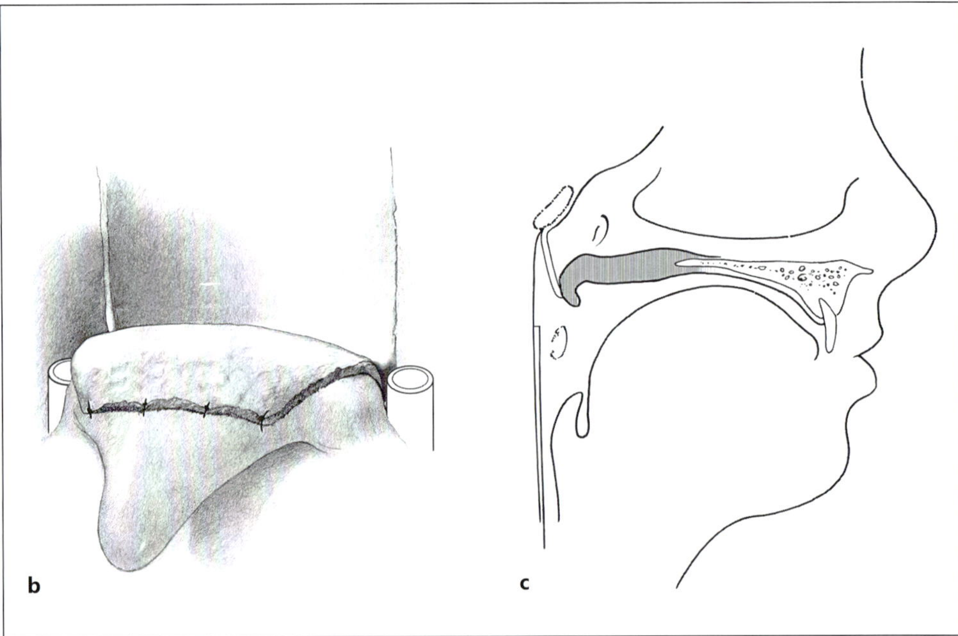

Fig. 6. The flap sutured in place. **a** All sutures placed with the endotracheal tubes in place. **b** The approximate location of the flap inset in relation to the edge of the soft palate. **c** Sagittal view of the flap inset.

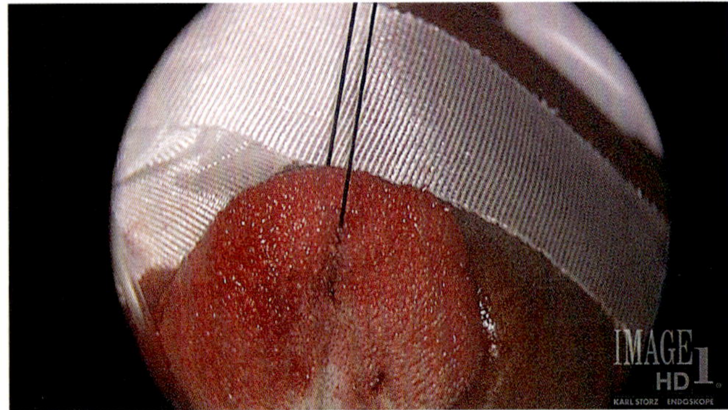

Fig. 7. Tongue suture placement.

Raol · Hartnick

Surgical Pearls

- Adequate hemostasis is vital in order to properly identify the surgical planes of dissection.
- The flap should be raised well into the nasopharynx because inadequate flap length can lead to tension on the closure and subsequent dehiscence.
- If large gaps are seen when checking the lateral ports after removal of the endotracheal tubes, the surgeon should not hesitate to place additional sutures. Persistent VPI due to overly generous lateral ports is more common than OSA due to excessive closure of lateral ports.
- Extubation should be performed with the patient completely awake, as obstruction may ensue if deep extubation is performed.

References

1 Schoenborn KWEJ: Ueber eine neue methode der staphylorrhaphie. Verh Dtsch Ges Chir 1875;4:235–239.
2 Padgett EC: The repair of cleft palates after unsuccessful operations. Arch Surg 1930;20:453–472.
3 Hogan VM: A clarification of the surgical goals in cleft palate speech and the introduction of the lateral port control (l.p.c.) pharyngeal flap. Cleft Palate J 1973;10:331–345.
4 Shprintzen RJ, Lewin ML, Croft CB, et al: A comprehensive study of pharyngeal flap surgery: tailor made flaps. Cleft Palate J 1979;16:46–55.
5 Sullivan SR, Marrinan EM, Mulliken JB: Pharyngeal flap outcomes in nonsyndromic children with repaired cleft palate and velopharyngeal insufficiency. Plast Reconstr Surg 2010;125:290–298.
6 Canady JW, Cable BB, Karnell MP, et al: Pharyngeal flap surgery: protocols, complications, and outcomes at the University of Iowa. Otolaryngol Head Neck Surg 2003;129:321–326.
7 Chegar BE, Shprintzen RJ, Curtis MS, et al: Pharyngeal flap and obstructive apnea: maximizing speech outcome while limiting complications. Arch Facial Plast Surg 2007;9:252–259.
8 Morris HL, Bardach J, Jones D, et al: Clinical results of pharyngeal flap surgery: the Iowa experience. Plast Reconstr Surg 1995;95:652–662.
9 Schmelzeisen R, Hausamen JE, Loebell E, et al: Long-term results following velopharyngoplasty with a cranially based pharyngeal flap. Plast Reconstr Surg 1992;90:774–778.
10 Witt PD, Myckatyn T, Marsh JL: Salvaging the failed pharyngoplasty: intervention outcome. Cleft Palate Craniofac J 1998;35:447–453.
11 Ysunza A, Garcia-Velasco M, Garcia-Garcia M, et al: Obstructive sleep apnea secondary to surgery for velopharyngeal insufficiency. Cleft Palate Craniofac J 1993;30:387–390.

Nikhila Raol, MD
Fellow, Pediatric Otolaryngology
Massachusetts Eye and Ear Infirmary
243 Charles St., Boston, MA 02114 (USA)
E-Mail nikhila_raol@meei.harvard.edu

Raol N, Hartnick CJ (eds): Surgery for Pediatric Velopharyngeal Insufficiency.
Adv Otorhinolaryngol. Basel, Karger, 2015, vol 76, pp 58–66 (DOI: 10.1159/000368019)

Sphincter Pharyngoplasty

Nikhila Raol · Christopher J. Hartnick

Pediatric Otolaryngology, Massachusetts Eye and Ear Infirmary, Boston, Mass., USA

Abstract

First described in 1950 by Hynes for patients with velopharyngeal insufficiency following cleft palate repair, the sphincter pharyngoplasty is a frequently used procedure for treating velopharyngeal insufficiency that rivals the pharyngeal flap in some centers as the most frequently used procedure. This technique is most effective for patients with good anterior-posterior motion but limited lateral wall motion. The primary aims of this chapter are to provide the clinician with indications for when to consider utilizing the sphincter pharyngoplasty and to give a stepwise description of how to perform the procedure.
© 2015 S. Karger AG, Basel

Introduction

Sphincter pharyngoplasty was initially described in 1950 by Hynes [1], who created bilateral salpingopharyngeal myomucosal flaps and rotated them 90°. These flaps were inset into the nasopharynx and sutured to the mucosa, where a transverse mucosal incision had been made below the tori tubarae. This procedure was recommended in children over 10 years of age to avoid the difficulty created by the presence of adenoid tissue.

In 1968, Orticochea [2] described a variation of this procedure, which is now a commonly used technique for sphincter pharyngoplasty, whether in its native form or with modifications. In this technique, bilateral myomucosal flaps were created using the posterior tonsillar pillars and the underlying palatopharyngeus muscles and were inset at the level of the oropharynx along the posterior pharyngeal wall. Orticochea later modified the location of the inset to be more superior, but Jackson's revision of the Hynes procedure in 1977 described the inset of the flaps at the level of the superior tonsillar pillars, which evolved to the current technique of suturing the flaps in a cephalad position in the nasopharynx.

Sie et al. [3] reviewed 24 cases of children with velopharyngeal insufficiency (VPI) who were treated with sphincter pharyngoplasty. The criteria for performance of this surgery included abnormal lateral wall motion (<4 on the Golding-Kushner scale) and no symptomatic evidence of sleep apnea. This group demonstrated a 62.5% (15/24) success rate, which was described as resolution of VPI without the need for revision surgery, improvement of nasometry scores, or resolution of hypernasality. Of note, 13% (3/24) of these patients developed hyponasality, which was not defined as surgical success. Of those who developed hyponasality, 66% (2/3) developed obstructive sleep apnea (OSA) symptoms, but none had evidence of OSA on polysomnography. Other studies that used resolution of VPI or need for further surgery as the definitions of success demonstrated success rates of over 80% for this procedure [4–6].

More recently, the notion of simultaneously addressing both the levator sling and lateral pharyngeal wall motion has been raised. Some surgeons have advocated the performance of sphincter pharyngoplasty in conjunction with a Furlow palatoplasty in the same procedure [7–10]. Carlisle et al. [9] compared the outcomes of 20 patients who underwent sphincter pharyngoplasty alone to those of 26 patients who underwent combined sphincter pharyngplasty and Furlow palatoplasty. In their study, the revision rate for those who underwent the combined procedure was only 4%, while the revision rate was 25% for the sphincter pharyngoplasty alone group. Most recently, Bohm et al. [11] compared pharyngeal flap, sphincter pharyngoplasty, and combined sphincter pharyngoplasty, and Furlow palatoplasty and the nasality severity score was used to compare the degree of VPI pre- and postoperatively. In this study, sphincter pharyngoplasty alone was used for patients with average nasality severity scores of 1.7 ± 0.92, while the pharyngeal flap and combined procedures were used for more severe VPI (2.24 ± 1.38 and 2.42 ± 1.29, respectively). The postoperative nasality severity scores were lower for both the pharyngeal flap group and the combined procedure group (0.61 ± 1.0 and 0.74 ± 1.03, respectively) compared to the sphincter pharyngoplasty alone group (0.9 ± 0.91). The pharyngeal flap was the only procedure that was complicated by nasopharyngeal stenosis, and the rates of OSA were 7.9% (3/38) for the pharyngeal flap, 10% (2/20) for sphincter pharyngoplasty, and 0% (0/38) for the combined procedure. Lastly, the surgical revision rates were 29, 20 and 8%, respectively [11]. These data suggest that sphincter pharyngoplasty is effective for VPI, but in cases where the anterior-posterior closure is also poor or the palate is short, the procedure may be increasingly effective when combined with a palatal lengthening procedure while still keeping the complication rate low. In these cases, the senior author allows nasal endoscopy and the intraoperative exam under anesthesia to dictate whether a combined procedure is indicated. In addition, it should be kept in mind that both sides of the velopharyngeal port are being addressed, so the risk of scarring of the soft palate to the posterior pharyngeal wall should not be overlooked.

Kilpatrick et al. [12] reviewed 36 patients who had undergone OSA following sphincter pharyngoplasty for various causes of VPI and demonstrated that no patients had apneic events or recorded desaturations in the immediate postoperative period, which led to their conclusion that outpatient sphincter pharyngoplasty should be considered. However, a 2012 review of 146 patients by Ettinger et al. [13] demonstrated an increase in OSA following sphincter pharyngoplasty, with the average apnea-hypopnea index value increasing from 3.1 to 8.4 episodes per hour. Previous adenotonsillectomy was predictive of the development of OSA following the procedure. In the senior author's experience, the risk of OSA is still present with a sphincter pharyngoplasty, but it is lower than the risk that accompanies pharyngeal flap surgery. Therefore, it is our practice to keep patients overnight following surgery to ensure that sleep apnea does not develop as a late complication.

Patient Evaluation

1. Office visit.
a. History, including genetic disorders, previous operations, cleft palate, etc.
b. Physical exam, including nasopharyngoscopy to evaluate the velopharyngeal closure pattern and evidence of medialized carotid arteries (see Chapter 3). A coronal closure pattern is most ideal for a sphincter pharyngoplasty.
2. Speech pathology evaluation, including fluoroscopy, if recommended by a speech pathologist (see Chapter 2).
3. Adjunct studies as needed, including cine MRI (see Chapter 4) and/or vascular imaging.

Indications

- VPI due to poor lateral wall motion, with good anterior-posterior motion and laterally located gaps upon velopharyngeal closure.
- VPI in patients with a circular closure pattern and contribution of Passavant's ridge where Passavant's ridge is shallow.
- Persistent VPI following other unsuccessful procedures.

Contraindications

- Pre-existing OSA. The tonsils should be evaluated for hypertrophy, and if needed, tonsillectomy should be performed. This is typically performed 6 weeks prior to primary surgery for VPI, but it has also been described as a simultaneous procedure.

- Midline/medial carotid vasculature (relative).
- Neuromuscular deficits causing immobile palate or clefts that are too wide to be repaired where an obturator/palatal lift is needed.

Anesthesia Considerations

- Midline endotracheal tube – an Oral Rae or armored tube is preferred to prevent 'kinking' of the tube during the course of the procedure.
- An in-depth discussion should be conducted with the anesthesiologist prior to the start of the procedure. It is imperative to relay the need for an awake extubation due to the possibility of a newly created obstruction in the nasopharynx. The patient should not be extubated during phase 2 and shouldbe completely awake prior to removing the tube. A tongue stitch should be placed prior to the end of the procedure for retraction in case of obstruction. A laryngeal mask airway should be kept nearby in the event of airway difficulty.

Materials

- Crowe-Davis mouth gag/tonsil set.
- Colorado tip Bovie.
- Multiple 4-0 Vicryl sutures on a small taper needle.

Set-Up

- A modified Rose position is used, with a generous shoulder roll for neck extension if the surgeon is seated for the procedure.
- The lateral and posterior pharyngeal walls should be observed for 30 seconds and then palpated to ensure the lack of pulsations, which would suggest abnormally located vasculature.
- The proposed posterior pharyngeal wall incisions are marked with either Gentian Violet or a surgical marker. Identical, superiorly based flaps should be marked bilaterally along the posterior tonsillar pillar, extending cephalad to the junction of the oropharynx and nasopharynx. Nearly the entire length of the posterior tonsillar pillar should be utilized (fig. 1).
- Local injection with lidocaine and 1:100,000 epinephrine should be performed along the proposed incision lines and the posterior pharyngeal wall at the junction of the oropharynx and the nasopharynx, with a wait time of 5–7 minutes to ensure adequate hemostasis.

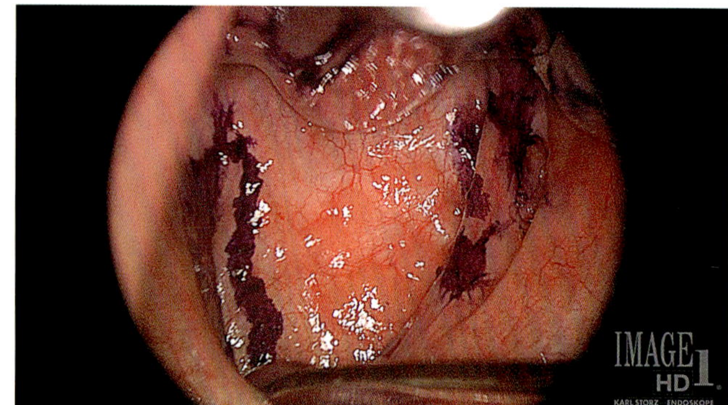

Fig. 1. The proposed incisions marked along the lateral posterior pharyngeal wall.

Procedure

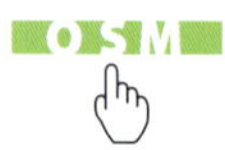

Sphincter Pharyngoplasty: Online supplementary video (for online supplementary material, see http://www.karger.com/Article/FullText/368019).

- A 3-sided incision is made on the right with a Colorado tip Bovie through the mucosa and muscle of the posterior pharyngeal wall until the prevertebral fascia is reached, leaving the tissue superiorly attached.
- The myomucosal flap is raised in an inferior to superior fashion into the nasopharynx with a Bovie and a peanut, using a pickup with teeth to gently grasp the flap (fig. 2). It is important to recognize the relationship between the posterior tonsillar pillar and the lateral and posterior pharyngeal walls.
  - o When a deep concavity is present behind the posterior pillar, the pillar itself should be displaced laterally when designing the flaps. By doing so, a true myomucosal flap can be raised as opposed to just a mucosal flap, which may happen when the posterior pillar alone is raised but is separated from the posterior and lateral walls by this deep groove.
- An identical, 3-sided incision is made on the left with a Colorado tip Bovie, and this flap is also raised in an inferior to superior fashion into the nasopharynx with a Bovie and a peanut, using a pickup with teeth to gently grasp the flap.
- The soft palate is then retracted superiorly with a Hurd retractor. The suction cautery on a setting of 20 is used to broadly demucosalize the posterior pharyngeal wall at the junction of the oropharynx and nasopharynx, thereby creating a surface for the inset of the flaps.
  - o A number of advantages exist to using the suction cautery instead of a knife to create the demucosalized surface. First, bleeding is kept to a minimum. Secondly, broad demucosalization can be obtained. Lastly, the flaps can be sutured to the raw surface instead of to the edge of a flap that has been elevated; this prevents bunching/redundancy of the tissue.
- The flaps are rotated 90°, and their position along the pharyngeal wall is approximated. If an extra flap length is present, the position of the flaps may be approximated

Raol · Hartnick

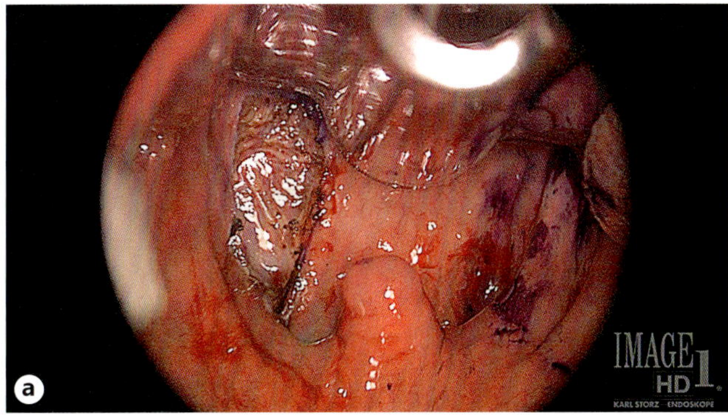

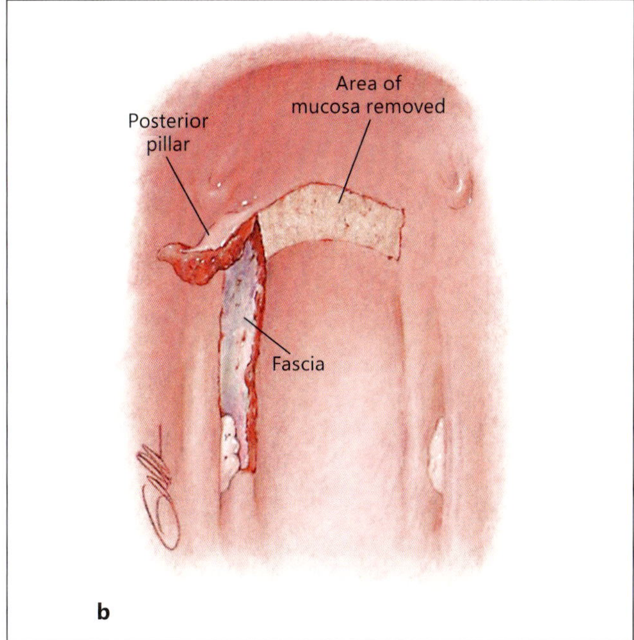

Fig. 2. Elevation of one flap. **a** Left side elevated, with a depth to the prevertebral fascia and elevation into the nasopharynx. **b** Right side elevated, with demonstration of the demucosalized region.

when they are adjacent and side-by-side to one another (fig. 3). Alternatively, the flap length may only be such that the flaps can meet at the midline. In this situation, the flaps should be approximated in an end-to-end fashion (fig. 4).

- The right-sided flap is then sutured to the edge of the demucosalized region of the posterior pharyngeal wall in one of the two configurations described above using 4-0 Vicryl sutures. The left-sided flap is then inset in the same fashion, and the two flaps are then sutured together, either side-by-side or end-to-end.
- A dental mirror is used to examine the central port to ensure a decreased distance between the soft palate and posterior pharyngeal wall.
- The posterior pharyngeal wall is closed on both the right and left sides using 4-0 Vicryl sutures with 2-3 simple interrupted stitches. Care should be taken to avoid bunching.

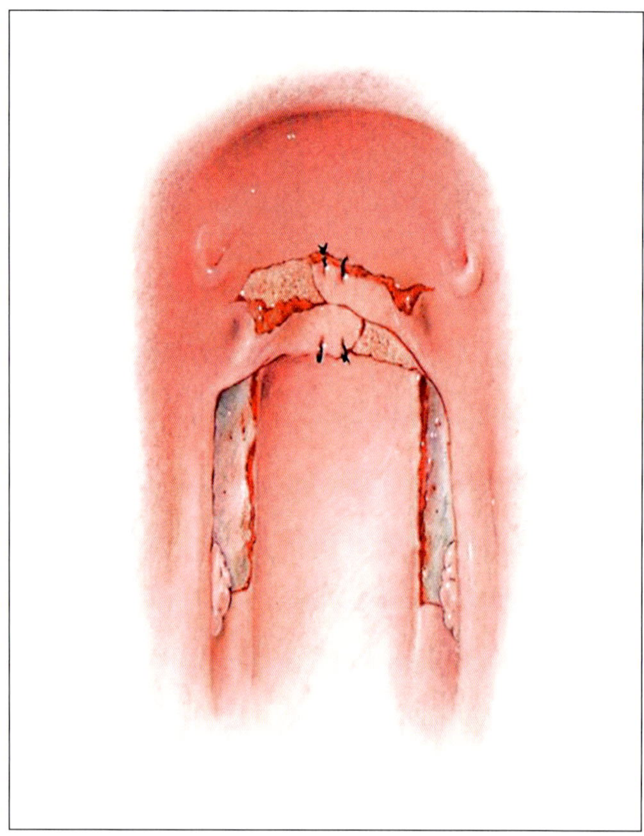

Fig. 3. A side-by-side inset of flaps.

- A 2-0 silk suture is then placed through the tongue as a retraction suture in case obstruction occurs postoperatively. This suture is taped to the cheek.
- The mouth gag is then carefully removed, and the patient is turned over to anesthesia for awake extubation.

Postoperative Care

- The patient should be monitored in a monitored/stepdown setting overnight for OSA.
- Care must be taken to prevent trauma to the repair. This might involve use of arm restraints during the postoperative period if the child has a propensity to put his/her fingers in the mouth. Additionally, the use of 'sippy' cups and straws should be avoided for approximately 3 weeks after surgery.
- Solid foods should be of a pureed consistency for 3 weeks following surgery. Foods such as breadcrumbs or crackers should be avoided to keep particles from getting trapped in the posterior pharyngeal wall.

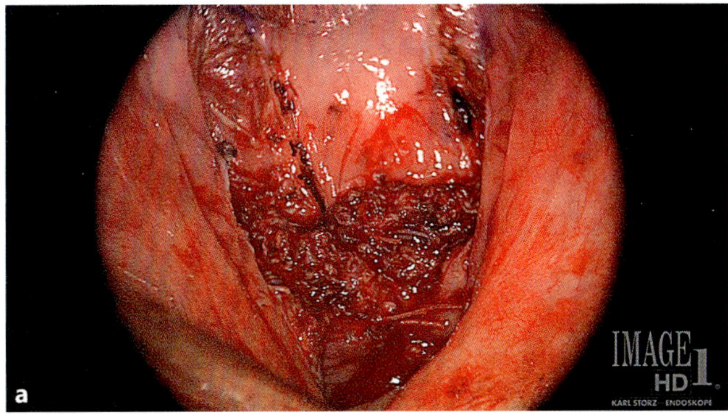

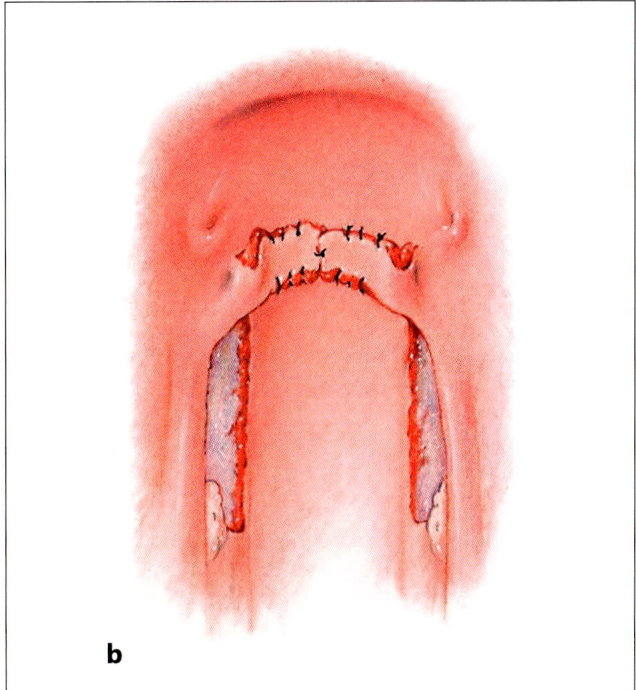

Fig. 4. An end-to-end inset of flaps, meeting in the midline. **a** An end-to-end inset shown in the patient. **b** Illustration of an end-to-end inset.

Surgical Pearls

- Adequate hemostasis is vital in order to properly identify the surgical planes of dissection.
- The relationship of the posterior tonsillar pillar to the posterior and lateral pharyngeal walls should be carefully noted. If a deep groove is noted behind the pillar, the pillar must be retracted laterally in order to create a strong myomucosal flap as opposed to a mucosa-only flap.
- The flaps should be raised well into the nasopharynx. In addition, extra attention should be given to complete and meticulous release of the lateral border of the flap,

as tethering here can prevent effective rotation, leading to tension on the closure and subsequent dehiscence.

- Use of suction cautery to demucosalize the posterior pharyngeal wall allows for broad demucosalization with excellent hemostasis.
- Nasal endoscopy and intraoperative exams should be carefully conducted to determine whether a combined procedure with a sphincter pharyngoplasty and a palatal lengthening procedure would be beneficial. These decisions should be made on an individual, case-by base basis.
- Extubation should be performed with the patient completely awake, as obstruction may ensue if deep extubation is performed. A tongue stitch will aid in relieving obstruction should it occur during/after extubation.

References

1 Hynes W: Pharyngoplasty by muscle transplantation. Br J Plast Surg 1950;3:128–135.
2 Orticochea M: Construction of a dynamic muscle sphincter in cleft palates. Plast Reconstr Surg 1968; 41:323–327.
3 Sie KC, Tampakopoulou DA, de Serres LM, et al: Sphincter pharyngoplasty: speech outcome and complications. Laryngoscope 1998;108:1211–1217.
4 Losken A, Williams JK, Burstein FD, et al: An outcome evaluation of sphincter pharyngoplasty for the management of velopharyngeal insufficiency. Plast Reconstr Surg 2003;112:1755–1761.
5 Pryor LS, Lehman J, Parker MG, et al: Outcomes in pharyngoplasty: a 10-year experience. Cleft Palate Craniofac J 2006;43:222–225.
6 Seagle MB, Mazaheri MK, Dixon-Wood VL, et al: Evaluation and treatment of velopharyngeal insufficiency: the University of Florida experience. Ann Plast Surg 2002;48:464–470.
7 Cheng N, Zhao M, Qi K, et al: A modified procedure for velopharyngeal sphincteroplasty in primary cleft palate repair and secondary velopharyngeal incompetence treatment and its preliminary results. J Plast Reconstr Aesthet Surg 2006;59:817–825.
8 Gosain AK, Arneja JS: Management of the black hole in velopharyngeal incompetence: combined use of a Furlow palatoplasty and sphincter pharyngoplasty. Plast Reconstr Surg 2007;119:1538–1545.
9 Carlisle MP, Sykes KJ, Singhal VK: Outcomes of sphincter pharyngoplasty and palatal lengthening for velopharyngeal insufficiency: a 10-year experience. Arch Otolaryngol Head Neck Surg 2011;137: 763–766.
10 Wojcicki P, Wojcicka K: Prospective evaluation of the outcome of velopharyngeal insufficiency therapy after pharyngeal flap, a sphincter pharyngoplasty, a double Z-plasty and simultaneous Orticochea and Furlow operations. J Plast Reconstr Aesthet Surg 2011;64:459–461.
11 Bohm LA, Padgitt N, Tibesar RJ, et al: Outcomes of combined Furlow palatoplasty and sphincter pharyngoplasty for velopharyngeal insufficiency. Otolaryngol Head Neck Surg 2014;150:216–221.
12 Kilpatrick LA, Kline RM, Hufnagle KE, et al: Postoperative management following sphincter pharyngoplasty. Otolaryngol Head Neck Surg 2010;142:582–585.
13 Ettinger RE, Oppenheimer AJ, Lau D, et al: Obstructive sleep apnea after dynamic sphincter pharyngoplasty. J Craniofac Surg 2012;23(Suppl 1):1974–1976.

Nikhila Raol, MD
Pediatric Otolaryngology
Massachusetts Eye and Ear Infirmary
243 Charles St., Boston, MA 02114 (USA)
E-Mail nikhila_raol@meei.harvard.edu

Raol N, Hartnick CJ (eds): Surgery for Pediatric Velopharyngeal Insufficiency.
Adv Otorhinolaryngol. Basel, Karger, 2015, vol 76, pp 67–73 (DOI: 10.1159/000368022)

Furlow Double-Opposing Z-Plasty

Nikhila Raol · Christopher J. Hartnick

Pediatric Otolaryngology, Massachusetts Eye and Ear Infirmary, Boston, Mass., USA

Abstract

First described in 1978 by Furlow for the repair of a cleft soft palate, the double-opposing z-plasty, also known as the Furlow palatoplasty, is an excellent procedure for repairing a submucous cleft. It is also useful in patients with touch closure who simply need lengthening of the soft palate and as an option for patients with anomalous carotid vasculature where pharyngeal flaps and sphincter pharyngoplasty are precarious. The primary aims of this chapter are to provide the clinician with indications for when to consider utilizing the Furlow palatoplasty and to give a stepwise description of how to perform the procedure.   © 2015 S. Karger AG, Basel

Introduction

The Furlow double-opposing z-plasty, initially described by Leonard Furlow in 1978 [1] for repairing a cleft soft palate, is a useful procedure for repairing velopharyngeal insufficiency (VPI) in patients with sagittal orientation of the levator veli palatini muscle. The goal of this surgery is to reorient the levator sling and lengthen the soft palate. Therefore, it serves as a useful tool for VPI patients with touch closure or a submucous cleft palate or for those with VPI following adenoidectomy (fig. 1).

Preoperative evaluation by nasopharyngoscopy and evaluation of the orientation of the levator sling and of the size of the velopharyngeal gap is essential when deciding whether a Furlow palatoplasty is the operation of choice. In a 2004 prospective study by Perkins et al. [2], 148 pediatric patients with mild to severe VPI underwent Furlow palatoplasty. Seventy-three percent of patients with mild VPI had resolution of symptoms, while only 13% of patients with severe VPI had resolution. Therefore, the algorithm used by these authors suggested the use of a

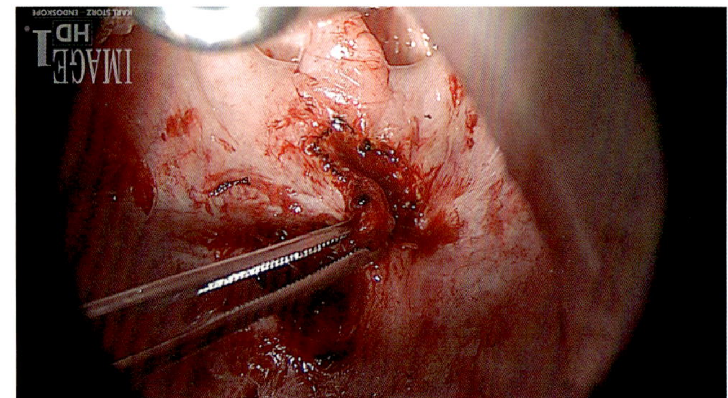

Fig. 4. Demonstration of the vector of closure of the oropharyngeal myomucosal flap.

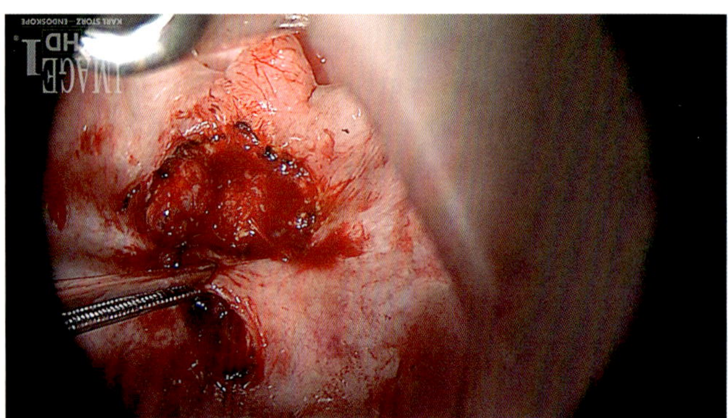

Fig. 5. Demonstration of the vector of closure of the oropharyngeal mucosal flap.

on the right side using a 4-0 Vicryl suture. A second suture is placed to secure the remainder of the oropharyngeal mucosal flap (fig. 4).

- The right-sided mucosal flap is then sutured to the corner of the cut edge of the oropharyngeal mucosa on the left side using a 4-0 Vicryl suture. Again, additional sutures are placed to secure the remainder of the flap to the oropharyngeal mucosa (fig. 5).
- The flaps of the second z-plasty are then sutured together (fig. 6).
- The mouth gag is then carefully removed, and the patient is turned over to anesthesia for awake extubation.

Postoperative Care

- The patient should be monitored overnight for edema and respiratory difficulty.
- Care must be taken to prevent trauma to the repair and might involve the use of arm restraints during the postoperative period if the child has a propensity to put his/her fingers in the mouth. Additionally, the use of 'sippy' cups and straws should be avoided for approximately 3 weeks after surgery.
- Solid foods should be of a pureed consistency for 3 weeks following surgery.

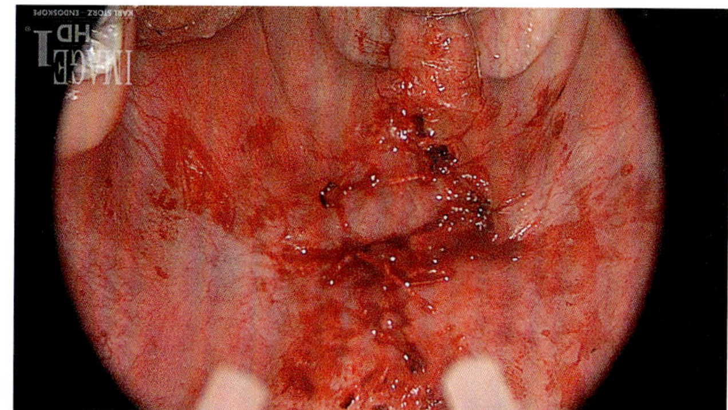

Fig. 6. A completely closed Furlow palatoplasty.

Surgical Pearls

- Adequate hemostasis is vital in order to properly identify the surgical planes of dissection.
- The myomucosal flap should always be the flap that is elevated from the side closest to the hard-soft palate junction toward the uvula, whether it is on the oropharyngeal or nasopharyngeal side. This will help plan incisions regardless of whether the surgeon is right- or left-handed.
- The mucosal flap should be handled very gently, as it can easily shred with trauma. Elevation with some minor salivary gland tissue on the posterior surface can help add some thickness to the flap while still leaving the muscle down.
- The nasopharyngeal-side z-plasty must be closed well to prevent fistula formation. Suturing the two flaps together is important to close the surgically created cleft.
- The vertical limb of the z incision should not extend to the hard/soft palate junction to decrease the likelihood of fistula formation.

References

1 Furlow LT Jr: Cleft palate repair by double opposing z-plasty. Plast Reconstr Surg 1986;78:724–736.
2 Perkins JA, Lewis CW, Gurss JS, Eblen LE, Sie KC: Furlow palatoplasty for management of velopharyngeal insufficiency: a prospective study of 148 consecutive patients. Plast Reconstr Surg 2005;116:72–80.
3 Rottgers SA, Ford M, Cray J, et al: An algorithm for application of Furlow palatoplasty to the treatment of velocardiofacial syndrome – associated velopharyngeal insufficiency. Ann Plast Surg 2011;66:479–484.
4 Sie KC, Tampakoupoulou DA, Sorom J, Gurss JS, Eblen LE: Results with Furlow palatoplasty in management of velopharyngeal insufficiency. Plast Reconstr Surg 2001;108:17–25.

Nikhila Raol, MD
Pediatric Otolaryngology
Massachusetts Eye and Ear Infirmary
243 Charles St., Boston, MA 02114 (USA)
E-Mail nikhila_raol@meei.harvard.edu

Raol N, Hartnick CJ (eds): Surgery for Pediatric Velopharyngeal Insufficiency.
Adv Otorhinolaryngol. Basel, Karger, 2015, vol 76, pp 74–80 (DOI: 10.1159/000368025)

Posterior Pharyngeal Wall Augmentation

Colleen F. Perez · Matthew T. Brigger

Naval Medical Center San Diego, Department of Otolaryngology – Head and Neck Surgery, San Diego, Calif., USA

Abstract

Posterior pharyngeal wall augmentation is a useful technique in selected patients with velopharyngeal insufficiency who have a small central velopharyngeal gap. Options for augmenting this region include using posterior pharyngeal wall flaps to create bulk and implanting various materials to fill in the central deficiency. Autologous and nonautologous implant materials are available and may be implanted through an incision or directly injected into the posterior pharyngeal wall. Previously described materials for implantation include cartilage, fat, fascia, silicone, acellular dermis, polytetrafluoroethylene, and calcium hydroxyapatite. Patient evaluation and surgical techniques for posterior pharyngeal wall augmentation are described.   © 2015 S. Karger AG, Basel

Introduction

Posterior pharyngeal wall augmentation is a surgical strategy to treat velopharyngeal insufficiency (VPI) by supplementing the posterior aspect of the velopharyngeal aperture. The goal is to improve soft palate contact with the posterior pharyngeal wall during velopharyngeal closure. The concept involves displacing the posterior pharyngeal wall anteriorly in such a way that it provides an easily reached contact point for the soft palate, allowing an adequate velopharyngeal seal and preventing nasal air escape during oral phonemes [1]. A variety of techniques have been described, with the classical approach being a superiorly based rolled pharyngeal flap. More recently, augmentation by direct implantation via an incision or injection into the posterior pharyngeal wall has been described. Autologous and nonautologous materials are

There is no potential conflict of interest, real or perceived, for any authors.

available and have been described, including cartilage, fat, fascia, silicone, acellular dermis, polytetrafluoroethylene, and calcium hydroxyapatite (CaHA) [2–6].

In the armamentarium of procedures to treat VPI, injection into the posterior pharyngeal wall is an easily performed procedure with low morbidity compared with more extensive pharyngeal procedures. The senior author prefers CaHA as an implant material due to its safety profile and efficacy over 24 months in properly selected patients [7]. The patients who benefit most from injection pharyngoplasty are those presenting with mild VPI and a small central velopharyngeal gap or touch closure that cannot withstand the fluctuating transvelar pressure of connected speech.

The rolled pharyngeal flap procedure, as classically described, results in morbidity similar to that of sphincter pharyngoplasty and a traditional superiorly based pharyngeal flap secured to the palate. The procedure is described below both for historical purposes and with the recognition that the technique may serve a role in treating select patients. In general, the technique has been abandoned at many centers due its morbidity, combined with reportedly poor outcomes compared with other techniques [8]. While the outcomes may be directly associated with patient selection, the morbidity of a rolled pharyngeal flap compared with the injection pharyngoplasty procedure is significantly greater. As such, the rolled flap procedure has been supplanted by injection pharyngoplasty as the augmentation procedure of choice at many centers.

Patient Evaluation

- All patients undergo evaluation by a speech and language pathologist to assess the severity and quality of VPI.
- A thorough review of preoperative nasendoscopy is performed to assess the location of air escape and to identify the ideal location for augmentation.
- Any history of velocardiofacial syndrome and other cardiac anomalies should be identified in order to assess the possibility of medialized carotid arteries.

Indications

- Mild VPI with touch closure or functional VPI during conversational speech.
- A small central velopharyngeal gap.
- Sagittal closure patterns benefit most from augmentation.

Contraindications

- Moderate to severe VPI.
- Large velopharyngeal gaps.

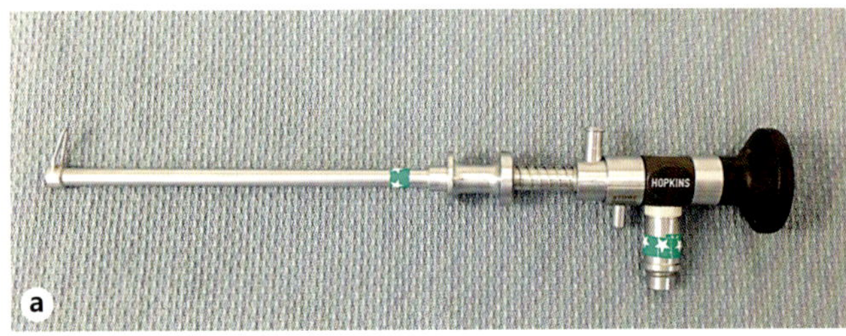

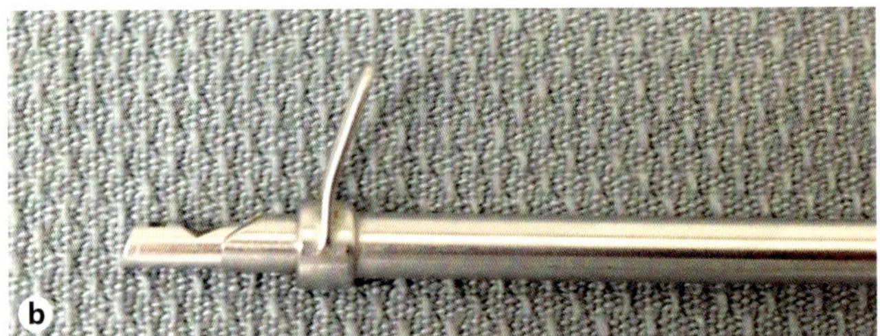

Fig. 1. a Image of 120-degree telescope with palate retractor. **b** Distal tip of endoscope with palate retractor engaged.

Materials

Injection Pharyngoplasty
- 120-degree endoscope with a palate retractor (fig. 1).
- Mouth gag.
- Long 25-gauge needle.
- Injection material.
- 0-degree endoscope if performing transnasal injection.

Set Up

Anesthesia Considerations
- General endotracheal anesthesia is required for young children.
- Local anesthesia may be used for transnasal injection pharyngoplasty in select older patients.

Procedure

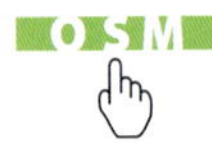

Injection Pharyngoplasty: Online supplementary video (for online supplementary material, see http://www.karger.com/Article/FullText/368025) and figure 2.
- The authors routinely administer perioperative antibiotics and steroids.
- Preoperative nasendoscopy is reviewed in the operating room to identify the location of the velopharyngeal gap to be injected with the desired implant material.

Perez · Brigger

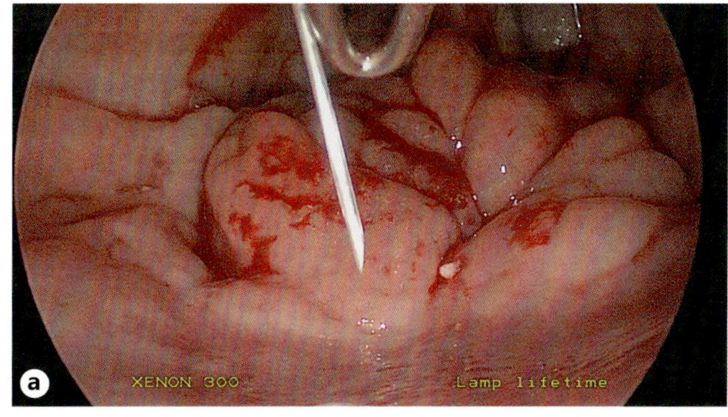

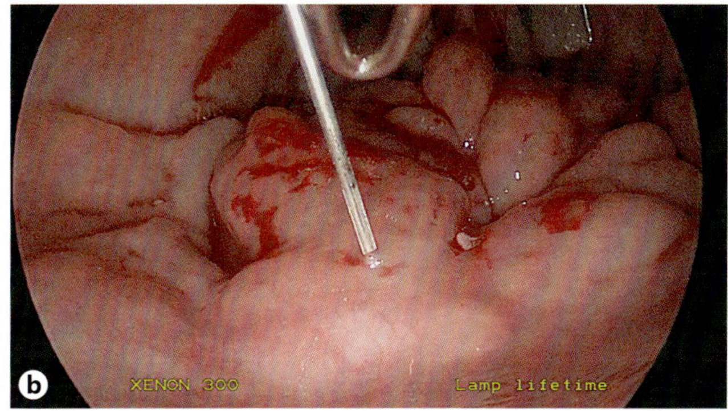

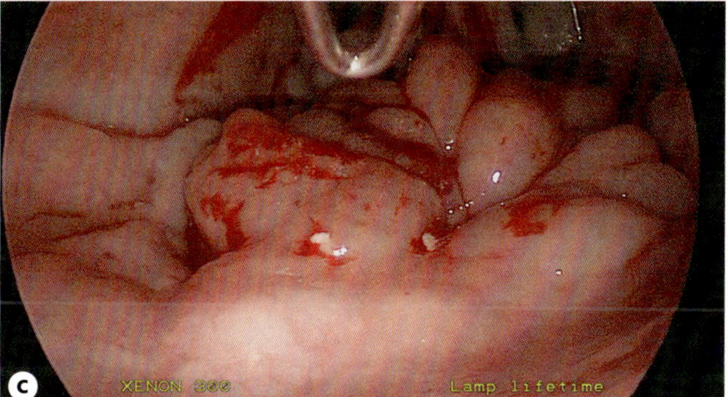

Fig. 2. a Intraoperative view of posterior pharyngeal wall prior to injection. **b** Intraoperative view of injection under direct visualization. **c** Intraoperative view of augmented posterior pharyngeal wall immediately after injection.

- The patient is positioned supine, and a shoulder roll is placed, as necessary, for neck extension.
- The mouth gag is inserted and the patient is placed into suspension.
- Visualize and palpate the posterior nasopharyngeal wall to identify anomalous vasculature.
- A 120-degree endoscope with a palate retractor is used for visualization (fig. 2a).
- The desired augmentation material is injected into the posterior pharyngeal wall target site by the transnasal or transoral route. The needle is inserted to the depth of bony contact and then withdrawn approximately 2 mm. The senior author

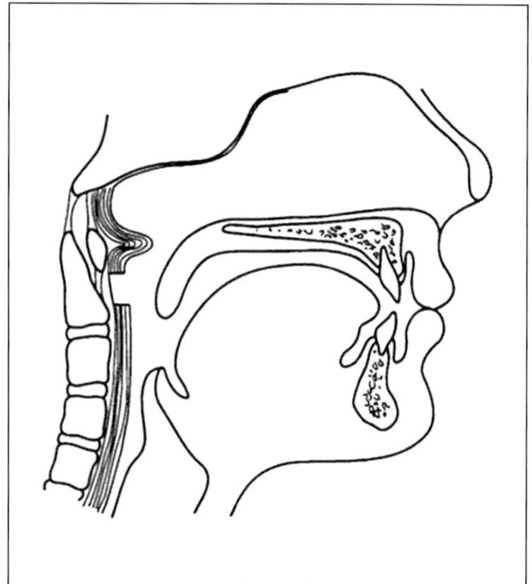

Fig. 3. Schematic of configuration of rolled pharyngeal flap (used with permission [9]).

prefers CaHA and generally injects 2–4 ml into the retropharyngeal space (fig. 2b).
- The injection of material is performed under direct visualization to provide adequate bulk, as determined by preoperative and intraoperative exams (fig. 2c).
- In select older patients undergoing transnasal injection, local anesthesia may first be performed with 4% lidocaine plus oxymetazoline. A 0-degree endoscope is placed through one nostril, and the needle for the injection material placed through the opposite nostril.

Superiorly Based Rolled Pharyngeal Flap (fig. 3)
- The patient is prepared as for the injection pharyngoplasty procedure and placed into the Rose position with a mouth gag.
- Similar to a traditional pharyngeal flap procedure (as described in Ch. 7), the width of the posterior pharyngeal flap is estimated as the distance between the posterior tonsillar pillars, with the inferior extent at the midpoint of the tonsillar fossa.
- The length of the flap is estimated as the distance from the free edge of the soft palate to the posterior pharyngeal wall.
- A local injection with 1% lidocaine plus 1:100,000 units epinephrine is performed at the planned incision sites.
- Lateral incisions are made down to the prevertebral fascia. Elevate the flap from inferior to superior, to the level of the natural velopharyngeal closure.
- Unlike a classical pharyngeal flap that is secured to the palate, the inferior edge of the flap is secured with 3-0 vicryl to the prevertebral fascia at the base of the flap. Thus, the flap is rolled onto itself, augmenting the posterior pharyngeal wall (fig. 3).
- Reapproximate the posterior pharyngeal wall defect with a 3-0 vicryl suture.

Perez·Brigger

Postoperative Care

- Patients undergoing injection pharyngoplasty may be discharged home on the day of surgery.
- Patients undergoing rolled pharyngeal flap surgery are observed overnight.
- Postoperative antibiotics are prescribed for 1 week.
- Patients return for postoperative evaluation at 1–2 weeks.
- Speech therapy may begin immediately following injection pharyngoplasty or in approximately 1 month following rolled pharyngeal flap surgery.

Pearls/Pitfalls

- The ideal candidate for posterior pharyngeal wall augmentation has mild VPI with a small central velopharyngeal gap and difficulty during connected speech.
- The morbidities associated with more extensive pharyngeal flap procedures are largely avoided with injection pharyngoplasty.
- A variety of autologous and nonautologous materials exist for injection pharyngoplasty.
- The rolled pharyngeal flap technique has largely been replaced by injection pharyngoplasty due to the ease of the technique and success of the procedure.
- Patients may be discharged home on the same day as injection pharyngoplasty.
- Persistent VPI may be improved with speech therapy; however, symptoms persisting beyond 3 months may necessitate more invasive surgical procedures.
- The potential exists for a foreign-body reaction, implant migration, or resorption that could lead to the need for further procedures.
- The presence of velocardiofacial syndrome or other cardiac anomalies should be determined in the patient's history and exam to evaluate possible anomalous vasculature. Preoperative imaging can be obtained to evaluate the possibility of medialized carotid arteries.

Financial Disclosure

None for all authors.
The views expressed in this article are those of the authors and do not necessarily reflect the official policy or position of the Department of the Army, the Department of the Navy, the Department of Defense, or the U.S. Government.

References

1 Perez CF, Brigger MT: Posterior pharyngeal wall augmentation; in Rogers DJ, Hartnick CJ, Hamdan US (eds): Video Atlas of Cleft Lip and Palate Surgery. San Diego, CA, Plural Pub., 2014, pp 291–294.

2 Willging JP, Cotton RT: Velopharyngeal insufficiency; in Bluestone CD, Stool SE, Alper CM (eds): Pediatric Otolaryngolog, 4th ed. Philadelphia, PA, Saunders, 2003, pp 1789–1799.

3 Lando RL: [Transplant of cadaveric cartilage into the posterior pharyngeal wall in treatment of cleft palate.] Stomatologiia (Mosk) 1950;4:38–39.

4 Bluestone CD, Musgrave RH, McWilliams BJ, Crozier PA: Teflon injection pharyngoplasty. Cleft Palate J 1968;5:19–22.

5 Blocksma R: Correction of velopharyngeal insufficiency by Silastic pharyngeal implant. Plast Reconstr Surg 1963;31:268–274.

6 Sipp JA, Ashland J, Hartnick CJ: Injection pharyngoplasty with calcium hydroxyapatite for treatment of velopalatal insufficiency. Arch Otolaryngol Head Neck Surg. 2008;134:268–271.

7 Brigger MT, Ashland JE, Hartnick CJ: Injection pharyngoplasty with calcium hydroxyapatite for velopharyngeal insufficiency: patient selection and technique. Arch Otolaryngol Head Neck Surg 2010;136: 666–670.

8 Witt PD, O'Daniel TG, Marsh JL, Grames LM, Muntz HR, Pilgram TK: Surgical management of velopharyngeal dysfunction: outcome analysis of autogenous posterior pharyngeal wall augmentation. Plast Reconstr Surg 1997;99:1287–1296; discussion 1297–1300.

9 Willging JP: Velopharyngeal Insufficiency; in Bluestone CD, Rosenfeld RM (eds): Surgical Atlas of Pediatric Otolaryngology. Hamilton, ON, BC Decker, 2002, p 416.

Matthew T. Brigger, MD, MPH, CDR, MC, USN
Naval Medical Center San Diego
Department of Otolaryngology – Head and Neck Surgery
34520 Bob Wilson Drive, San Diego, CA 92134 (USA)
E-Mail matt.brigger@alumni.vanderbilt.edu

Raol N, Hartnick CJ (eds): Surgery for Pediatric Velopharyngeal Insufficiency.
Adv Otorhinolaryngol. Basel, Karger, 2015, vol 76, pp 81–85 (DOI: 10.1159/000368032)

Persistent Velopharyngeal Insufficiency

J. Paul Willging[a, b]

[a]Division of Pediatric Otolaryngology – Head and Neck Surgery, Cincinnati Children's Hospital Medical Center,
Cincinnati, Ohio, [b]Department of Otolaryngology – Head and Neck Surgery, University of Cincinnati College of
Medicine, Cincinnati, Ohio, USA

Abstract

This chapter outlines the management of patients who have failed initial surgical correction of velopharyngeal insufficiency. Clinical judgment is required to determine the most appropriate revision
option for each patient.   © 2015 S. Karger AG, Basel

Background

In most pediatric patients, surgical correction of velopharyngeal insufficiency (VPI)
results in normal or improved resonance. A small percentage (5%) of patients,
however, continue to have abnormal resonance or nasal air emission postoperatively,
despite undergoing a 3- to 6-month period of speech therapy aimed at maximizing
the functional results of surgery. If a successful outcome is not achieved within this
timeframe, nasopharyngoscopy should be performed to visualize the adequacy of
velopharyngeal closure and determine the etiology of the persistent problem.

The otolaryngologist should assess the surgical repair in regard to its location
within the velopharyngeal sphincter. A pharyngeal flap that is too low allows air to
escape around it, and a port that is too large cannot be completely closed by medial
movement of the lateral pharyngeal walls. Asymmetric lateral wall motion or a flap
that is skewed to one side may result in air leakage on just one side of the
velopharyngeal sphincter. Failure of a sphincter pharyngoplasty may result in air
escape if the lateral pharyngeal walls were not medialized sufficiently or if the
posterior pharyngeal wall was not sufficiently augmented by the transposition flaps.
In cases of posterior wall augmentation, nasal escape can occur if the injected

material is not in the plane of closure or if the volume of injected material was inadequate.

Once the cause of persistent VPI has been determined, a management plan can be developed.

Indications for Revision Procedures

- Clinicians must be cognizant of the fact that in most instances, any of the surgical techniques discussed below may be a viable option for revision.
- Selection of a specific technique is largely based on clinical judgment, considering the needs of each individual patient.

Revision Procedures

Options for Patients Who Have Undergone Pharyngeal Flap Surgery
- Redo flap.
- Injection pharyngoplasty.
- Reposition flap with or without mucosal advancement.

Redo Flap (Lining the Flap)
When a second pharyngeal flap is needed, the clinician must be cognizant of why the initial flap failed. If infection caused the initial flap to dehisce, the patient should be kept on antibiotics after the revision to minimize the risk of infection. If flap failure is attributed to insufficient anchoring into the soft palate, the pocket in the soft palate should be made large enough to accept the flap. Consideration should also be given to the number and size of the sutures being used to prevent dehiscence from occurring a second time.

Occasionally, a pharyngeal flap contracts and fibroses to the point at which there is only a small band remaining in the pharyngeal sphincter. In this setting, the lateral ports are large and unamenable to narrowing procedures. Replacing the pharyngeal flap may be the only option for improving velopharyngeal function. To minimize the risk of flap fibrosis recurring, the undersurface of the flap is lined to reduce secondary intention healing of the raised flap.

Procedure
- Raise the pharyngeal flap as described in chapter 7.
- Divide the palate at the midline, extending the incision from the free margin of the soft palate halfway to the hard palate.
- Elevate the nasopharyngeal mucosa to the free edge of the soft palate.
- Incise the nasopharyngeal mucosa to create a mucosal flap that is pedicled on the free margin of the soft palate.

- Inset the pharyngeal flap into the velum as discussed in chapter 7.
- Tack the nasopharyngeal mucosal flaps to the raw undersurface of the flap.
- Close the muscular layer of the palate.
- Close the oral mucosa of the palate.

Injection Pharyngoplasty

The inability to close the lateral ports during connected speech may be caused by several different problems: (1) the flap may be low and out of the plane of closure, (2) the flap may be narrow, or (3) the mobility of the lateral walls may be insufficient to allow closure. Injection pharyngoplasty with Deflux (a dextranomer/hyaluronic acid copolymer) may be used to modify the size of the lateral ports; however, this material is not approved by the Food and Drug Administration for use in the treatment of VPI and is used primarily in the treatment of pediatric vesicoureteral reflux. Port Narrowing Injection: Online supplementary video 1 (for all online supplementary material, see http://www.karger.com/Article/FullText/368032).

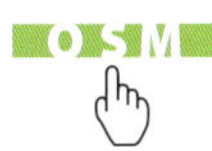

  Endoscopy of the patient allows identification of the degree of closure of the velopharyngeal ports. The area of air escape (i.e. right, left, bilateral) can be determined, and the size of the gap can be visualized. It is essential to have this information available intraoperatively during the revision procedure.

Procedure
- The patient is suspended in the Rose position.
- Next, 8 Fr suction catheters are passed through the nose, passed through each port, and brought out through the mouth to retract the palate and apply tension to the ports.
- The ports can often be viewed without the use of a mirror.
- Deflux is placed into an oropharyngeal injector and must be transferred to a 1-ml tuberculin syringe in order to fit into this device.
- Deflux is injected submucosally to narrow the port at the site(s) determined during the preoperative endoscopic evaluation.
- In view of the absorption of some of the injected Deflux volume, a slight overcorrection should be made in the volume of injected material.

Repositioning the Flap With or Without Mucosal Advancement
- If the pharyngeal flap is low (i.e. below the plane of velopharyngeal closure), air will escape around the flap. Port Narrowing Flap Revision: Online supplementary video 2 (for all online supplementary material, see http://www.karger.com/Article/FullText/368032).

Procedure
- The patient is suspended in the Rose position.
- Next, 8 Fr suction catheters are passed through the nose, passed through each port, and brought out through the mouth to retract the palate and apply tension to the ports.

- An incision is made laterally and inferior to the flap, down to the prevertebral fascia. The superior attachment of the flap is not incised.
- The flap can be pushed superiorly to occupy its proper position within the velopharyngeal sphincter.
- The raw surface created inferior to the flap requires closure.
- If the lateral ports are too large, the mucosa within these ports can be advanced to close the defect and simultaneously narrow the port(s).
- The mucosal advancement is sewn into the recipient bed to close the mucosal defect and limit downward migration of the pharyngeal flap.
- If the lateral ports do not need to be narrowed, the mucosa of the posterior pharyngeal wall can be advanced superiorly to close the defect.
- An alternative is to reposition the pharyngeal flap and narrow the lateral ports with Deflux injections.

Options for Patients Who Have Undergone Sphincter Pharyngoplasty
- Redo the sphincter pharyngoplasty.
- Injection pharyngoplasty.
- Deconstruct the sphincter pharyngoplasty and convert to a pharyngeal flap.

A second sphincter pharyngoplasty is performed similarly to the original procedure described in chapter 8. The transposition flaps are inset into the previous insertion site. This further augments the posterior pharyngeal wall and narrows the lateral aspect of the velopharyngeal port.

If a previous sphincter pharyngoplasty results in a narrow gap that continues to allow air to escape, the velopharyngeal port can be narrowed with injection pharyngoplasty. Deflux can be injected into the port in the area of deficiency to allow the port to close during connected speech.

It is generally not possible to place a pharyngeal flap into the residual port remaining after a sphincter pharyngoplasty. Complete nasopharyngeal stenosis would develop if a flap were to be inserted. However, if the velopharyngeal port following a sphincter pharyngoplasty is so large that a flap is deemed necessary, the sphincteroplasty must be deconstructed. This is done by making lateral incisions in the original sphincter pharyngoplasty, which will open the velopharyngeal sphincter area. Following deconstruction, resonance worsens. Revision can be completed once the area has healed, generally after a period of 6 weeks. A pharyngeal flap can then be inserted as described in chapter 7.

Options for Patients Who Have Undergone Posterior Pharyngeal Wall Augmentation
- Further augmentation.
- Pharyngeal flap.
- Sphincter pharyngoplasty.

If a posterior pharyngeal wall augmentation procedure fails to correct VPI, additional injection pharyngoplasty procedures can be performed. The site of air escape must be visualized so that Deflux can be properly injected, allowing improvement in velopharyngeal closure.

If multiple revisions via injection pharyngoplasty have been performed to no avail, an alternative surgical option should be considered. In this circumstance, pharyngeal flap surgery or a sphincter pharyngoplasty can be performed as described in chapters 7 and 8, respectively.

Pearls and Pitfalls

- Regardless of the surgical technique used to correct VPI, a small percentage of patients will continue to have abnormal resonance or nasal air emission after initial surgical correction.
- Although nasal resonance may improve postoperatively, improvement is not equivalent to normalization.
- Input from the patient's family is critical in assessing the impact of abnormal resonance on speech intelligibility and in making a decision as to whether the patient should undergo surgical revision.
- Any of the surgical revision techniques discussed in this chapter may be a viable option for revision.

Selection of a specific technique requires sound clinical judgment, considering the cause of persistent VPI and the needs of each individual patient.

J. Paul Willging, MD
Division of Pediatric Otolaryngology – Head and Neck Surgery
Cincinnati Children's Hospital Medical Center
3333 Burnet Avenue, MLC 2018, Cincinnati, OH 45229 (USA)

palate; this retains bulk on the soft palate, which maximizes the ability to maintain velopharyngeal closure while improving the airway.

- The resulting defect on the posterior pharyngeal wall is left open to granulate.

Pearls and Pitfalls

Increasing the Size of the Ports
- There is usually a specific site within the port that causes the obstruction. Attention to that specific area will allow the port to spring open when it is divided.
- Minimal modification to the flap itself is required to open the port.
- Enlarging the velopharyngeal port(s) may cause abnormal resonance or the development of nasal air emission if the moving lateral wall cannot make contact with the flap during connected speech.

Flap Takedown
- If a flap has been in position for a long period of time prior to takedown, resonance often remains normal.
- Flap takedown does not always normalize the airway, as tongue base obstruction or hypopharyngeal collapse may also lead to OSA.

J. Paul Willging, MD
Division of Pediatric Otolaryngology – Head and Neck Surgery
Cincinnati Children's Hospital Medical Center
3333 Burnet Avenue, MLC 2018, Cincinnati, OH 45229 (USA)

Author Index

Subject Index